# Palliative Care
## A patient-centered approach

*Edited by*
GEOFFREY MITCHELL
Associate Professor of General Practice
University of Queensland, Australia

Radcliffe Publishing
Oxford • New York

**Radcliffe Publishing Ltd**
18 Marcham Road
Abingdon
Oxon OX14 1AA
United Kingdom

www.radcliffe-oxford.com
Electronic catalogue and worldwide online ordering facility.

© 2008 Geoffrey Mitchell

Geoffrey Mitchell has asserted his right under the Copyright, Designs and Patents Act 1998 to be identified as the author of this work.

All rights reserved. No part of this publication may be reproduced, stored in a retrieval system or transmitted, in any form or by any means, electronic, mechanical, photocopying, recording or otherwise, without the prior permission of the copyright owner.

British Library Cataloguing in Publication Data

A catalogue record for this book is available from the British Library.

ISBN-13: 978 1 85775 739 2

Typeset by Egan Reid, Auckland, New Zealand
Printed and bound by TJI Digital, Padstow, Cornwall, UK

**Library
University of Texas
at San Antonio**

# Contents

# Series editors' introduction

The strength of medicine in curing many infectious diseases and some of the chronic diseases has also led to a key weakness. Some believe that medicine has abdicated its caring role and, in doing so, has not only alienated the public to some extent, but also failed to uphold its promise to 'do no harm'. One hears many stories of patients who have been technically cured but feel ill or who feel ill but for which no satisfactory diagnosis is possible. In focusing so much attention on the nature of the disease, medicine has neglected the person who suffers the disease. Redressing this 20th century phenomenon required a new definition of medicine's role for the 21st century. A new clinical method, which has been developed during the 1980s and 1990s, has attempted to correct the flaw, to regain the balance between curing and caring. It is called a Patient-Centered Clinical Method and has been described and illustrated in *Patient-Centered Medicine: Transforming the Clinical Method* (Stewart *et al.*, 2003).[1] In the 2003 book, conceptual, educational and research issues were elucidated in detail. The patient-centered conceptual framework from that book is used as the structure for each book in the Series introduced here; it consists of six interactive components to be considered in every patient-practitioner interaction.

The first component is to assess the two modes of ill health: disease and illness. In addition to assessing the disease process, the clinician explores the patient's illness experience. Specifically, the practitioner considers how the patient feels about being ill, what the patient's ideas are about the illness, what impact the illness is having on the patient's functioning, and what he or she expects from the clinician.

The second component is an integration of the concepts of disease and illness with an understanding of the whole person. This includes an awareness of the patient's position in the life cycle and the proximal and distal contexts in which they live.

The third component of the method is the mutual task of finding common ground between the patient and the practitioner. This consists of three key areas:

mutually defining the problem; mutually defining the goals of management/ treatment; and mutually exploring the roles to be assumed by the patient and the practitioner.

The fourth component is to use each visit as an opportunity for prevention and health promotion. The fifth component takes into consideration that each encounter with the patient should be used to develop the helping relationship; the trust and respect that evolves in the relationship will have an impact on other components of the method. The sixth component requires that, throughout the process, the practitioner is realistic in terms of time, availability of resources and the role of collaborative teamwork in patient care.

However, there is a gap between the description of the clinical method and its application in practice. The series of books, presented here, attempts to bridge that gap. Written by international leaders in their field, the series represents clinical explications of the patient-centered clinical method. Each volume deals with a common and challenging problem faced by practitioners. In each book, current thinking is organized in a similar way, reinforcing and illustrating the patient-centered clinical method. The common format begins with a description of the burden of illness, followed by chapters on the illness experience, the disease, the whole person, the patient-practitioner relationship and finding common ground including current therapeutics.

The book series is international, to date representing Norway, Canada, New Zealand, the USA, England and Scotland. This is a testament to the universality of the values and concepts inherent in the patient-centered clinical method. We feel that an international definition of patient-centered practice is being established and is represented in this book series.

The vigor of any clinical method is proven in the extent to which it is applicable in the clinical setting. It is anticipated that this series will inform further development of the clinical method and move thinking forward in this important aspect of medicine.

Moira Stewart PhD
Judith Belle Brown PhD
Thomas R Freeman MD, CCFP
September 2007

## References

1 Stewart, M., Brown J.B., Weston, W.W., McWhinney, I.R., McWilliam, C.L. & Freeman, T.R. (2003) *Patient-Centered Medicine Transforming the Clinical Method*. (2e) Oxford, UK, Radcliffe Publishing.

# About the editor

**Geoffrey Mitchell** is Associate Professor in the Discipline of General Practice, University of Queensland. He has also been awarded an Australian Government Primary Health Care Senior Research Fellowship. He has dual specialist qualifications in general practice and palliative medicine, and was awarded a Doctor of Philosophy (PhD) for work on the use of case conferences as a means of involving and improving the skills of general practitioners (GPs). He maintains a general practice in Ipswich, Australia.

He has been involved in general practice education and research for over 20 years. He played a central role in developing palliative care services in his community, an interest which expanded to supporting the maintenance of palliative care skills in GPs across Australia. This has resulted in the production of the first national guidelines for palliative care, and research into the factors that promote and inhibit GPs maintaining involvement in palliative care. He has also conducted research into the GP management of other complex problems, notably attention deficit hyperactivity disorder, and clinical research methodology, particularly drug trials using single-patient trial methodology.

# List of contributors

**Amy Abernethy** is an Assistant Professor of Medicine at Duke University School of Medicine, Assistant Professor of Nursing at Duke University, and Adjunct Associate Lecturer at Flinders University in South Australia. She is a faculty member of both the Duke Clinical Research Institute and the Duke Comprehensive Cancer Center Cancer Control Program, and a Senior Fellow of the Duke Center for Clinical Health Policy Research. Dr Abernethy's research focuses on conducting high-quality clinical trials that generate evidence-based solutions for common problems in palliative care such as cancer pain, dyspnea, and health service delivery models.

**Stephen Barclay** is Macmillan Cancer Support Post-Doctoral Research Fellow, Honorary Consultant Physician in Palliative Medicine, and Specialty Director for Palliative Medicine in the Cambridge University Medical School, England. He is also Honorary Senior Lecturer in Primary Palliative Care at the Department of Palliative Care Policy and Rehabilitation at King's College Medical School, London. He is a GP in a practice in Cambridge, and visiting clinician to the Arthur Rank House Hospice in Cambridge. He has extensive clinical and research experience in primary palliative care.

**David Currow** is Chief Executive Officer of Cancer Australia, the national agency charged with the development and implementation of cancer policy in Australia. He is a medical oncologist, and is also Professor of Palliative and Supportive Services at Flinders University in Adelaide, South Australia. He received his medical degree from the University of Newcastle and is a Foundation Fellow of the Australasian Chapter of Palliative Medicine and Fellow of the Royal Australasian College of Physicians. He is President of the Clinical Oncological Society of Australia, and immediate past president of Palliative Care, Australia. His research interests include clinical research into palliative care symptoms, public health and health policy approaches to palliative care, and the translation of evidence into practice.

**Richard Harding** is Lecturer in Palliative Care, King's College, University of London, England. He originally read social anthropology and has a Master's in Social Policy and Social Work Studies. His PhD addressed informal carers in palliative care. His clinical experience includes human immunodeficiency virus (HIV) and palliative care management, acute adult health hospital social work, and community care management. He also designs and delivers community-based group work focused on behavioural change. His academic interests in palliative care are informal carers, HIV, palliative care provision in Africa, and the evaluation of complex interventions. His broader interests are in behavioural interventions and HIV prevention. His current work is focused on palliative care in Sub-Saharan Africa.

**Janet Hardy** is Professor of Palliative Medicine at the University of Queensland, Brisbane, Australia. She graduated from Auckland Medical School and trained in medical oncology at Auckland Hospital. After achieving Doctor of Medicine, she took up a position as Senior Registrar in Medical Oncology at the Royal Marsden Hospital in London. She worked closely with the palliative care team at the Royal Marsden and in 1991 was offered the position of locum consultant in palliative care. She was subsequently appointed to a substantive consultant post as Head of the Department of Palliative Medicine and Head of Research. In 2003, she took up the position of Director of Palliative Care at the Mater Health Services Brisbane. She maintains an active interest in palliative care research and is now the Clinical Research Programme Leader for the Centre for Palliative Care Research and Education. Her major research interests are in the clinical development of new analgesics and analgesic formulations, the management of cancer-related nausea and vomiting, and facilitating research in palliative care. Her mission is to improve the evidence base on which the practice of palliative care is founded.

**Irene Higginson** is Professor and Head of Department, Palliative Care, Policy and Rehabilitation, at King's College, University of London, England. She qualified in medicine from Nottingham University and has worked in wide-ranging medical and university positions, including radiotherapy and oncology, in-patient and home hospice care, the Department of Health (England), and various universities. Her last post was as Senior Lecturer/Consultant at the London School of Hygiene and Tropical Medicine and Director of Research and Development at Kensington and Chelsea and Westminster Health Authority. She has been at King's as Professor and Head of Department since October 1996. Her research interests and publications are in the areas of quality of life and outcome measurements, evaluation of palliative care (especially new services and interventions), epidemiology, clinical audit, effectiveness, psychosocial factors and care, symptom assessment, cachexia/anorexia, and elderly care.

**Jenny Hynson** is the Pediatrician of the Victorian Paediatric Palliative Care Program. She is the recipient of an Australian Government Palliative Care Research Fellowship for a project to improve the evidence base of pediatric palliative care. Her expertise has contributed to national palliative care guidelines.

**Allan Kellehear** is Professor of Sociology in the Department of Social and Policy Sciences. He was born and educated in Sydney, Australia, and holds a PhD in sociology from the University of New South Wales. From 1998 to 2006 he was Professor of Palliative Care and Director, Palliative Care Unit, School of Public Health, of La Trobe University in Melbourne, Australia. During that time he also served as the 2003–04 Visiting Professor of Australian Studies at the University of Tokyo, Japan. He joined the University of Bath and teaches a program in Death and Society. He is co-editor with Dr Glennys Howarth of *Mortality*, the international journal of interdisciplinary studies in death and dying. His current research interests include the history, sociology and social psychology of dying; mystical, religious and altered states associated with dying and bereavement; public health policies, service sector development and models of care for dying; the sociology of health and illness; health promotion, community development and social ecology; and qualitative and unobtrusive research methodology.

**Jonathon Koffman** is Lecturer in Palliative Care at King's College, University of London, England. He has a Bachelor of Science (BSc) in Social Administration and a Master of Science (MSc) in Sociology with Special Reference to Medicine from Royal Holloway and Bedford New College. Jonathon's previous work experience involved health services research and health services commissioning for a number of health authorities. He is now Lecturer in Palliative Care and Course Co-ordinator for the inter-professional Postgraduate Certificate, Diploma and MSc in Palliative Care, run in collaboration with St. Christopher's Hospice. His research interests include the end-of-life experiences of black and minority ethnic groups, social exclusion, qualitative research, and palliative care education. He has published in the areas of culture and ethnicity, older people, needs assessment, social exclusion and palliative care, palliative care education, HIV and acquired immune deficiency syndrome (AIDS), as well as mental health and homelessness.

**Geoffrey Mitchell** is Associate Professor of General Practice at the University of Queensland, Australia, and is an Australian Primary Health Care Research

Evaluation and Development Senior Research Fellow. His PhD was a study of the effects of formal specialist–general practitioner case conferences on the quality of life of dying people. His research has been in the maintenance and improvement of clinical palliative care skills in family practice, the interface between specialists and family practitioners, the primary care of other chronic and complex conditions, and clinical research methodology, particularly drug trials using single-patient trial methodology. He maintains a clinical general practice.

**Judith Murray** is a Senior Lecturer in Psychology at the University of Queensland, Australia, Director of the Master of Counselling course. She initially gained a Bachelor of Arts (BA) and Diploma of Education in Mathematics and History. She completed first-class honours in psychology and later a PhD, which focused on community interventions with bereaved families. She has nationally recognized expertise in loss, grief and bereavement, and has taught and written extensively on these topics. Major themes of research have been in the area of reactions to bereavement and other situations of loss, and the development and evaluation of interventions to enhance mental well-being. Her current research interests are in the assessment and management of spiritual issues in palliative care.

**David and Clare Seamark** are GPs in Honiton, rural Devon, England. David is Honorary Senior Clinical Research Fellow of the Peninsula Medical School of the Universities of Exeter and Plymouth, England. Together they conduct qualitative, clinical and health services research in a range of conditions. In this context their research is in patient and carer experiences of advanced non-malignant disease, and of the degree to which the health system is responsive to the needs of palliative care patients.

**Patsy Yates** is Professor and Research Director of the School of Nursing, and Head of the Centre for Palliative Care Research and Education at Queensland University of Technology, Brisbane, Australia. She has extensive clinical, educational and research experience in cancer and palliative care, and for several years has held a joint academic–clinical appointment with the Division of Oncology at Royal Brisbane Hospital. Her areas of expertise are pain and symptom management, supportive care for people with cancer, and educational strategies for cancer palliative care practice. She is currently undertaking funded studies evaluating supportive interventions for people experiencing pain, breathlessness and fatigue. She is immediate past Chairperson for the Cancer Nurses' Society of Australia, and member of the Board of Trustees for the International Society of Nurses in Cancer Care. She is also a member of the Medical and Scientific Committee of the Cancer Council Australia.

# Acknowledgements

It has been a pleasure writing and editing this book. I am grateful to Professors Moira Stewart, Judith Belle Brown and Thomas Freeman from The University of Western Ontario for the opportunity to do so, and for their expert guidance. Thanks to Andrea Burt for her prompt and cheerful editorial assistance.

To my co-authors, thanks for offering your willing co-operation. It has been an honour to collaborate with such esteemed colleagues.

Much of this work was conducted while on sabbatical leave from the Discipline of General Practice at the University of Queensland, Australia. I would like to thank my colleagues, particularly Drs Marie-Louise Dick, Deborah Askew and Jenny Doust, for sharing the load in my absence. I would also like to express grateful thanks to John and Eleanor Swift, who hosted me and my family several times whilst visiting Canada during the book's development.

Finally, thanks to my patients and colleagues at Limestone Medical Centre, Ipswich, for teaching me so much and giving so much.

*To Anne, for her constant love and support,
and to Anna and Sam, for being fantastic kids.*

*I am truly blessed.*

# CHAPTER 1

# Introduction

*GEOFFREY MITCHELL*

## Overview

Death will come to us all – for some quickly, and for others over weeks, months or years. Where the latter course occurs, the final stages of life are a time of declining physical capacity and increasing reliance on others. Increasing symptoms, physical dependence, and uncertainty about their personal future and that of their loved ones are some aspects of a fearsome and sometimes dark journey.

The care of palliative care patients encapsulates all facets of good family practice: if a doctor does family practice well, he or she will do palliative care well. However, while palliative care can be relatively straightforward, problems can arise that are beyond the skill of a generalist. Now that palliative care specialist teams exist there is backup advice and support for most family practitioners. But having specialist teams available in most locations is not a reason to cede all palliative care to them. Too many people die, and specialist teams cannot cope with them all. It is in everyone's interest for family practitioners to be competent in this area.

Death is unfamiliar territory for many in the Western world. Not many people have seen a dead person or watched someone die. When dying does occur, it occurs outside the context of the person's normal life – frequently in hospitals or other care facilities.

In the middle part of the 20th century death was seen as medical failure. Spectacular medical and social advances had robbed formerly killer diseases of their potency, and most people started living to old age. When treatments failed to arrest the progress of diseases, health practitioners found they did not have the wherewithal to manage a patient's death. In the last days, dying patients would be placed in a single room, sometimes not even visited by healthcare staff. It was as if the health profession could not face the fact that they could not control the disease, so it was best not acknowledged at all. Needless to say, symptom control was poor, and the physical suffering that many endured reinforced the mood of the day – that dying was repulsive and death was to be feared.

A paradigm shift occurred in the 1960s, which swung the pendulum away from complete dependence on high-technology medicine towards a more integrated approach. In a general sense this movement began when Ralph Nader challenged consumers to ask questions about the goods and services they received, rather than simply assume that the providers knew best. With respect to dying, twin influences arose through two remarkable women studying dying patients from diverse points of view. A young Cicely Saunders commenced work as a nurse, then social worker, then finally as a doctor. She was the first to study the process of dying systematically – in particular, the management of pain in dying people. In time she developed a completely new institution to care for dying people and to provide an environment where scientific study of the process could be carried out. From that beginning in 1966 has grown a new medical specialty, palliative medicine. At around the same time, sociologist Elisabeth Kübler-Ross deliberately studied the experiences of dying patients. Her seminal book, *On Death and Dying*,[1] forced society to look at how it understood death, and how it should understand the experience of, and relate to, the dying.

Out of these advances has arisen the palliative care movement. It is no accident that palliative care is frequently described as a movement. At the time it was both a medical advance and a social advance. It was led by lay people questioning healthcare and in particular the care of dying people. At the same time, doctors and academics willing to question the status quo put enormous effort into providing a scientific basis to end-of-life care. The result has been the global development of a new way of providing care for the dying – palliative care. The World Health Organization's definition of palliative care highlights the rigour that the discipline of palliative care should demonstrate, while promoting the expectation that healthcare will create an environment and systems that pay homage to the innate human experience that is dying.

A quiet revolution also took place in family practice (also known as general practice or primary healthcare in different parts of the world) at around the same time. Michael Balint used psychotherapeutic supervision of British GPs to create a better understanding of the profound impact the relationship between doctor and patient has on patient outcomes.[2] He termed this phenomenon 'doctor as drug' to highlight the power of this effect.

In-depth study of the power of the family practice consultation enlarged our understanding of how this power can be harnessed to the benefit of the patient.

Concepts like Pendleton *et al.*'s 'Tasks of the consultation', a term coined in the 1980s, now drive clinical family practice by introducing the concept that satisfactory outcomes for a consultation require a multifaceted approach.[3]

Stewart *et al.* have brought all these strands together in what they term the 'patient-centered clinical method'.[4] Where Pendleton *et al.*'s model is somewhat doctor-centered (i.e. what the doctor should achieve in the consultation), Stewart and co-authors place the patient at the center of their model, requiring the doctor to apply their knowledge of a disease process to the patient, and to pay attention to the many facets of the patient's experience and that of those around them.

## What is the patient-centered clinical method?

Figure 1 pictorially represents the patient-centered method of clinical practice. The method consists of six interactive components.

1. Initially the *disease* is considered, but at the same time the patient's *experience of being ill with the disease* has to be explored. The two are inextricably inter-woven and therefore have to be understood as a single entity comprising related paradigms.

2. Understanding the whole person is the component that seeks to *place the disease/illness entity into context*; that is, to understand its place in the whole person. This means giving consideration to three questions:

   ▶ How does the disease/illness entity affect the person?
   ▶ How does the person interact with those elements of their immediate environment, and vice versa? Immediate environment is described as *proximal context*, and includes those parts of the environment with which the person has regular, close contact. This includes their family, work, school and other close social networks.
   ▶ How does the wider environment influence this interaction? The wider environment will include community, culture, health and political systems, socio-historical systems, geography, the media, the environment, and so on. This is termed the *distal context*.

3. The third component of the patient-centered method is termed *finding common ground*. Patient and clinician reach a mutual understanding and agreement on the nature of the problems, the goals of management, and who will be responsible for what.

The final three parts of the model relate to strategies and understanding of the patient–doctor relationship that will improve the performance of the whole system.

4. The first is the desirability of undertaking *broader health-promoting* and *illness-prevention tasks* within the consultation. Most patients visit a GP or family

practitioner at least once a year. These doctors have unparalleled opportunities to influence the health-enhancing behavior of that individual.

5. The second is to have *an understanding of the patient–doctor relationship* in order to *enhance it*. It is a relationship that should be valued greatly by practitioners, and an understanding of the investment that patients put into this relationship should make doctors very mindful of the way they exercise their part in it. Their use of the relationship can enhance the power of the consultation for everyone's good, but it can also do irreparable harm.

6. Finally, the practitioner needs to assess *what can be realistically achieved* to assist the patient. Practical limits to the time and skills of the practitioner need to be acknowledged by both patient and practitioner. The possibilities of enhancing the power of the health encounter through working in teams need to be recognized and, if possible, implemented. The wise stewardship of resources also needs to be taken into account.

Each of these elements of the patient-centered model is examined in detail in its own chapter.

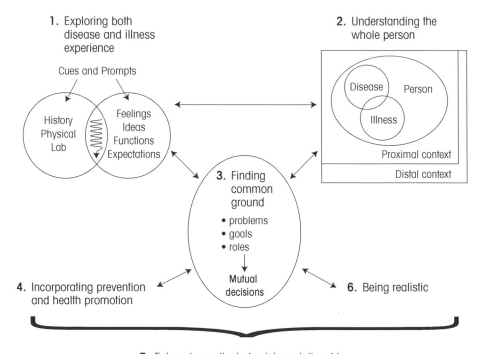

**FIGURE 1** The patient-centered clinical method: six interactive components

## The aims of this book

This book applies the patient-centered method to the practice of palliative care. There are significant overlaps between palliative care and family or general practice. Both are centered on the patient, and both recognize the essence of a multidisciplinary or multifaceted approach to patient care. Both expect high-quality, evidence-based approaches to care, and both disciplines are currently working hard to accumulate that evidence. Finally, most of palliative care will be conducted in the community, with family or GPs undertaking a large share of the medical care of the patient and the family.

This book brings a fresh perspective to the subject by presenting it through a patient-centered lens. It presents a model and a method of care, but not every nuance of the subject. World experts in their fields examine palliative care from points of view as diverse as epidemiology, palliative medicine, nursing, behavioral science, sociology and health promotion. The model and method bring these points of view together. Books that present in-depth material on medical techniques, drug doses and the like are freely available. This sort of information is described briefly in the text, but the detail can be easily sourced elsewhere.

We hope this will be an important resource for clinicians and educators in the medical, nursing and allied health professions. It provides valuable information for policy-makers and administrators by presenting an intellectual framework within which patient care policy and procedures can be formulated and enacted. We trust you will enjoy the book, and will find ways in your own practice to use the patient-centered clinical method to enhance the care of your patients.

## References

1  Kübler-Ross E. *On Death and Dying.* London: Tavistock; 1970.
2  Balint M. *The Doctor, His Patient and the Illness.* New York: International Universities Press; 1972.
3  Pendleton D, Schofield T, Tate P, *et al. The Consultation: an approach to learning and teaching.* Oxford: Oxford University Press; 1984.
4  Stewart MA, Brown JB, Weston WW, *et al. Patient-centered Medicine: transforming the clinical method.* 2nd ed. Oxford: Radcliffe Medical; 2003.

# CHAPTER 2

# Palliative care: the magnitude of the problem

*JONATHAN KOFFMAN, RICHARD HARDING, IRENE HIGGINSON*

## Introduction: the universal right to care at the end of life

> We emerge deserving of little credit; we who are capable of ignoring the conditions that make muted people suffer. The dissatisfied dead cannot noise abroad the negligence they have experienced.[1]

Nearly 40 years ago in this statement John Hinton drew attention to the deficiencies that were evident in the care offered to many patients with advanced disease and their families. While we have witnessed a growing understanding of the palliative care needs of patients and their families and an acceptance that death is universal – which, *de facto*, makes it a universal public health concern – the actual provision of care has remained in part woefully inadequate.

In recent years, both in the UK and elsewhere, questions are being asked about how much palliative care we need, by whom, where, and at what cost, given that accessible and good-quality care towards the end of life must be recognized as a basic human right.

> Everyone has the right to . . . security in the event of sickness, disability, widowhood, old age or other lack of livelihood in circumstances beyond his [or her] control. *Article 25, United Nations Universal Declaration of Human Rights 2001*

Currently, however, we lack many of the critical pieces of information to answer all of these questions adequately, although there is broad agreement based on local and national epidemiological surveys,[2,3] government reports and World Health Organization (WHO) data[4,5] that the palliative services currently available from a range of providers are inadequate to meet some existing, and the rapidly growing, health and social care needs of the world's citizens with advanced disease.

In this chapter we explore the concept and various approaches used to determine the magnitude of palliative care requirements of patients with advanced disease and their families in a local population. We then draw on current evidence, primarily but not exclusively from the UK and the USA, on how specialist and generic services have met the palliative care needs of some underserved and overlooked population groups. These include informal caregivers of patients with advanced disease, the poor, the very elderly, people with learning disabilities, black and minority ethnic communities, asylum seekers and refugees, drug users, and those within the penal system.

Although this chapter has limited itself to these disenfranchised population groups, other marginalized patient groups or sectors of the population are not immune. They include those who are homeless or live in fragile accommodation, travelers, and those who abuse alcohol. However, little attention – and therefore published research – has focused on either their met or unmet palliative care needs, a testimony to their social distance from the mainstream. The complex needs of patients with non-malignant disease and their informal carers are eloquently described in detail elsewhere.[6] We conclude by offering some innovative strategies that have been offered to meet the palliative care needs of these population groups.

## What exactly is need?

According to Soper, 'There can be few concepts so frequently invoked and yet so little analyzed as that of human needs'.[7] Other contributions to the definitions of need come from the fields of sociology, epidemiology, health economics and public health, as well as from clinicians.

Most doctors would consider need in terms of the healthcare services they can supply. Patients may have a different view, because need incorporates the wider social and environmental determinants of health, such as deprivation, housing, diet, education and employment. This wider definition allows us to look beyond the confines of the medical model based on health services to the wider influences on health. It is for this reason that in 1972 Bradshaw distinguished four types of need, which are summarized in Box 2.1. Note that Box 2.1 suggests that need, demand and supply are of equal size. There is little evidence to suggest that this is actually the case in many countries.

**BOX 2.1**  Need: who decides and how?

Need can be:
- what the individual feels they want (felt need)
- what the individual demands (expressed need)
- what a professional thinks the individual wants (normative need)
- how we compare with others' areas or situations (comparative need).

Source: Bradshaw J, 1972[8]

These distinctions raise questions about who determines need (professionals, politicians or the general public?), the influences of education and the media in raising awareness about health problems, and the cultural effects on need. Social and cultural factors have an enormous impact on levels of morbidity and on the expression of health needs (*see* Box 2.2).

**BOX 2.2**  What influences need?

Need is influenced by:
- knowledge of what might be available and possible, derived from friends, family, culture, media, the internet, health and social care professionals, etc.
- developments in knowledge
- expectations from service providers
- information about what works
- ability to express need – some people are more eloquent or able to express need than others
- effect of peers and information on professionals
- what can be described and operationalized.

Source: Higginson and Goodwin, 2001[9]

The most pragmatic definition of need for our purposes is 'the ability to benefit from health care', originally developed by the National Health Service (NHS) Executive in the UK and now used in several countries.[10]

## Assessing need

To assess the palliative care needs of a local population, three strategies can be adopted: the epidemiological, the comparative and the corporate.

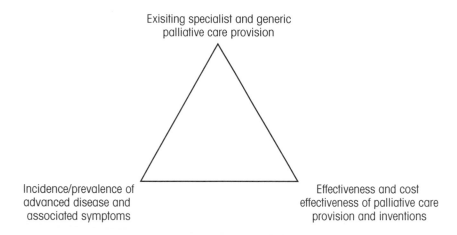

**FIGURE 2.1** Components of health needs assessment

## The epidemiological approach

The epidemiological approach makes use of local cause-specific mortality in diseases that are *likely* to benefit from palliative care services, and then relates this to the type and frequency of symptoms experienced by patients suffering from these diseases. It reviews the effectiveness and cost effectiveness of care using local, national, and international evidence. Lastly, it compares these with the patterns of locally available specialist and generic services to determine how well need is being met (Figure 2.1).[11]

### Epidemiologically based palliative care needs assessment for patients with advanced disease

In an attempt to assist the process of providing comprehensive information on the extent of local palliative care needs, an epidemiologically based needs assessment for palliative and terminal care has been produced for the UK NHS Executive.[12] The document provides standard definitions of palliative and terminal care and uses national and local data on the incidence and prevalence of cancer and likely symptoms to estimate the numbers of patients and families needing palliative care. The actual local numbers of patients dying from cancer and other diseases are available from the Office of National Statistics or local health authorities. Family doctors may also have data from their own records, or access to *ad hoc* surveys.

Table 2.1 shows the number of deaths within a population during a typical year for the most common causes in England. There are roughly equal numbers of men and women who died, and the numbers would be roughly constant over the years. A typical age distribution for England and Wales would be: < 15 years <1%; 16–35 years 3%; 36–64 years 19%; 65–74 years 21%; 75+ years 56%. Applying the prevalence of symptoms to this population gives estimates of the number of people with different problems and the size of the population needing care.

**TABLE 2.1** Number of deaths in the population during one year for the most common causes

|  | MEN | WOMEN | TOTAL |
|---|---|---|---|
| **Cause of death** | | | |
| Neoplasms* | 1464 | 1341 | 2805 |
| Circulatory system | 2429 | 2624 | 5053 |
| Respiratory system | 595 | 626 | 1211 |
| Chronic liver and cirrhosis | 34 | 26 | 60 |
| Nervous system and sense organs* | 88 | 88 | 176 |
| Senile and pre-senile organic conditions | 22 | 22 | 44 |
| Endocrine, nutritional, metabolic, immunity | 187 | 123 | 310 |
| **Total of these diseases** | **4819** | **4850** | **9669** |
| **Total of causes of death** | **5356** | **5644** | **11 000** |

Notes: total population = 1 million, because of small numbers for some categories in 10 000; deaths in those aged under 28 days excluded.

\* For breakdown of main group see below.

| **Cause of death** | | | |
|---|---|---|---|
| Neoplasms include: | | | |
| lip, oral, pharynx, larynx | 41 | 34 | 75 |
| digestive and peritoneum | 449 | 339 | 788 |
| trachea, bronchus, lung | 394 | 291 | 685 |
| female breast | 0 | 255 | 255 |
| genitourinary | 243 | 178 | 421 |
| lymphatic and hematopoietic | 154 | 54 | 208 |
| other, unspecified | 7 | 7 | 14 |
| Nervous system and sense organs include: | | | |
| Parkinson's disease | 37 | 28 | 65 |
| multiple sclerosis | 1 | 1 | 2 |
| meningitis | 4 | 4 | 8 |

Source: Higginson, 1997[2]

In a population of 10 000 people (e.g. a typical UK primary care group practice), national estimates suggest that there are approximately 28 cancer deaths per year, many of whom would have a period of advancing progressive disease, during which palliative care would be appropriate. The estimates of prevalence of symptoms and problems are based on population and other studies of patients with advanced disease and their families. Applying the population estimates to the 28 patients who would die from cancer suggests that there would be 24 with pain, 13 with breathlessness, 14 with vomiting or feeling sick, 20 with loss of appetite and nine where the patient (and seven where the family) had severe anxiety or worries which were seriously affecting their daily life and concentration (*see* Table 2.2).

**TABLE 2.2** Cancer patients: prevalence of problems (per 10 000 population)

| SYMPTOM | % WITH SYMPTOM IN LAST YEAR OF LIFE* | ESTIMATED NUMBER IN EACH YEAR |
|---|---|---|
| Pain | 84 | 24 |
| Trouble with breathing | 47 | 13 |
| Vomiting or feeling sick | 51 | 14 |
| Sleeplessness | 51 | 14 |
| Mental confusion | 33 | 9 |
| Depression | 38 | 11 |
| Loss of appetite | 71 | 20 |
| Constipation | 47 | 13 |
| Bedsores | 28 | 8 |
| Loss of bladder control | 37 | 10 |
| Loss of bowel control | 25 | 7 |
| Unpleasant smell | 19 | 5 |
| | | |
| Severe family anxiety/worries | 33 | 9 |
| Severe patient anxiety/worries | 25 | 7 |
| Total deaths from cancer | | 28 |

* Symptoms as per the Cartwright and Seale study, based on a random sample of deaths and using the reports of bereaved carers.[13,14]

Notes: Anxiety as per references 15–18. Patients usually have several symptoms.

Source: Higginson, 1997[2]

The studies of Cartwright and Seale used random samples of bereaved carers as informants. This has the advantage of providing data on all cancer deaths, and not just the groups of patients receiving specialist care, or included in special studies. Such patients might be different from the 'average', which has resulted in their referral to a particular service. For example, they may have had more severe symptoms, or might be different because they were known to services.

However, using bereaved carers as informants may be flawed because the information represents the carer's perspective, which is coloured by their own grief rather than the patient's actual view.[19] Few studies have examined this, but it may be that families overestimate symptoms or dichotomize their views during bereavement. Even so, the prevalence of many symptoms (such as pain) are roughly similar in the studies of Cartwright and Seale as in other large surveys. This suggests that although on an individual basis reports may vary, when a population is considered as a whole the results are reasonable. Families are part of the unit of care, so their views have validity in this context.

Current levels of use of specialist palliative care services can also be used to estimate need. In England, studies have estimated that between 15 and 25% of those dying of cancer received inpatient hospice care, with between 25 and 65% receiving input from a support team or Macmillan nurse. Applying these figures to a typical general practice population would suggest that each year seven to eighteen cancer patients require support team care, and four to seven require inpatient hospice care (*see* Table 2.3). Some patients will obviously require both services, and some may be admitted to a hospice two or more times. Estimates of average service use nationally do not necessarily indicate that these levels of use are correct. This is considered in greater detail in the evidence section, later in the chapter.

**TABLE 2.3** Cancer patients: need for specialist palliative services based on national and regional estimates of use (per 10 000 population)*

|  | NUMBER OF ADULTS | % |
| --- | --- | --- |
| Deaths from cancer in one year: | 28 | |
| Needing support team | 7–18 | 25–65 |
| Needing inpatient hospice care | 4–7 | 15–25 |
| * Studies used include references 13–18 and 20–23. | | |

Source: Higginson, 1997[2]

### Epidemiological data: need among non-cancer patients and their families

As for cancer patients, estimates of the prevalence of symptoms and other problems experienced by non-cancer patients and their families can be applied to determine the number of people with these problems in the last year of life (*see* Table 2.4).

The number of people affected is more than double those for cancer.[24] Primary care contributes significantly toward the care of these patients and their families. In many of the illnesses it is more difficult to prognosticate, because the illness is sometimes acute, sometimes progressive and sometimes chronic. Traditionally, specialist palliative care services have concentrated on people with cancer, but this is changing. Such services see their role as increasingly providing expert symptom control and psychosocial advice and care for people with other illnesses – in those instances where they have the skills to help. As specialist palliative care services move towards providing more home care, respite care and short admissions to attend to symptom or other problems, they may become increasingly able to help with this aspect of care. Therefore, estimates of need based on the current patterns of use of specialist palliative care services (*see* Table 2.5) are likely to be inaccurate; although they may give an indication of those patients who need especial attention.

**TABLE 2.4** Patients with non-cancer progressive illness: prevalence of problems (per 10 000 population)

| SYMPTOM | % WITH SYMPTOM IN LAST YEAR OF LIFE* | ESTIMATED NUMBER IN EACH YEAR |
|---|---|---|
| Pain | 67 | 46 |
| Trouble with breathing | 49 | 34 |
| Vomiting or feeling sick | 27 | 18 |
| Sleeplessness | 36 | 25 |
| Mental confusion | 38 | 26 |
| Depression | 36 | 25 |
| Loss of appetite | 38 | 26 |
| Constipation | 32 | 22 |
| Bedsores | 14 | 10 |
| Loss of bladder control | 33 | 23 |
| Loss of bowel control | 22 | 15 |
| Unpleasant smell | 13 | 9 |
| | | |
| Severe family anxiety/worries | 33 | 22 |
| Severe patient anxiety/worries | 25 | 16 |
| Total deaths from other causes, excluding accidents, injury and suicide, and causes very unlikely to have a palliative period | | 68 |

\* As per the Cartwright and Seale study, based on a random sample of deaths and using the reports of bereaved carers. [13,14]

Notes: Anxiety as per references 15–18. Patients usually have several symptoms.

Source: Higginson, 1997[2]

## Need during bereavement

The primary care team is often the first point of contact for a bereaved person. For every person who dies there may be one or more bereaved carers who will have physical, emotional, social and spiritual changes as a result of their loss. This will apply for both chronic and acute deaths.

Grief is known to have a marked effect on mortality and morbidity. Mor *et al.* found that when age, sex and prior health were controlled for, bereaved spouses were at increased risk of physician visits, hospitalization, use of anti-anxiety medication and increased alcohol use compared with national averages.[28] In a study of bereaved older adults, Norris and Murrell found that bereavement was followed by increased 'psychological distress'.[29] All these effects will result in needs for care and support during bereavement, although the extent of this in the primary care setting is not well researched.

**TABLE 2.5** Patients with progressive non-malignant diseases: need for specialist palliative services based on local studies of use or need (per 10000 population)*

|  | NUMBER OF ADULTS | % |
| --- | --- | --- |
| Deaths in one year | 69 | |
| Needing support team | 4–14 | 0.5–1 times numbers of cancer patients needing care |
| Needing inpatient palliative care | 2–7 | 0.5–1 times numbers of cancer patients needing care |
| * Studies used include references 25–27. | | |

Source: Higginson, 1997[2]

## Comparative and corporate approaches to palliative care needs assessment

The comparative needs assessment approach examines levels of service utilization rather than disease categories. A common approach is to compare and contrast the local levels of activity against national averages so that areas of specialist practice can be examined for obvious disparities in equity of provision.[2] But there are a number of difficulties in this approach. The main limitation is that it does not assess unmet need, which must then be evaluated by other methods. Comparing a locality with other regions is problematic, not least because populations can vary considerably in terms of demographic make-up, ethnicity and social deprivation. Lastly, the corporate needs assessment approach involves a structured collection of the knowledge and views of local informants on healthcare services and unmet needs. Valuable information is often available from a wide range of parties; for example, managers who work in primary care settings, family doctors and other healthcare professionals, and (importantly) patients and their families.[30]

The corporate approach is essential if policies to meet unmet need are to be sensitive to local circumstances. There are, nevertheless, caveats in adopting this approach. Those undertaking the exercise must be aware of bias and the politics of vested interests.[31] Also, the assessment may produce a multitude of needs, although criteria can be used to prioritize these needs (e.g. the importance of a problem in terms of frequency or severity, the evidence of effectiveness of interventions, or the feasibility for change). Needs assessments that do not include sufficient attention to policy implementation will become little more than academic or public relations exercises.

## Palliative care services and unmet need: what is the evidence?

The concept of equity of access to healthcare is a central objective of many healthcare systems throughout the world. In the early 1970s, Julian Tudor Hart coined the phrase 'inverse care law' to describe his observation that those who were in the greatest apparent need of care often had the worst access to healthcare provision.[32] Since that time, although a growing body of research evidence has accumulated quantifying the problem,[33–36] the aspiration of making healthcare available to all has remained elusive.

This has been no less of a challenge for those who require care at the end of life.[37–39] This may be due to palliative care services previously being developed largely based on assumptions about patient need from healthcare professionals' points of view.[40] In recent years in the UK the commitment to tackle health inequalities among disenfranchised population groups has been harnessed under the wing of 'social exclusion', a relatively new term in the UK policy debate to describe an old problem.[41] It includes poverty and low income, but is broader and addresses some of the wider causes and consequences of social deprivation. The UK Government has defined social exclusion as:

> . . . a shorthand term for what can happen when people or areas suffer from a combination of linked problems such as unemployment, poor skills, low incomes, poor housing, high crime, bad health and family breakdown.[42]

Social exclusion is something that can happen to anyone. However, some people from certain backgrounds are more likely to suffer.

Although palliative care has become more prominent within the mainstream NHS during the last decade, it has still been very slow to meet the complex needs of certain patients and the family members who could benefit from it. Below we have focused on the available evidence of access to palliative care for poor and other disenfranchised population groups (*see* Figure 2.2). Our list of groups is admittedly restricted, and we emphasize that other vulnerable sectors of the society may fare as badly.

## Informal caregivers

The palliative 'total care' model aims to offer high-quality care not just to the patients but also to their families and informal carers, who may be relatives, partners, friends and members of their wider community. The tasks they perform may be broad, including one or more of practical, emotional and physical care.[43]

Informal palliative care has significant implications for primary care, as higher rates of physical illness are reported among the ranks of recently bereaved informal carers,[28] and emotional strain during caring has been identified as a mortality risk factor among elderly spousal carers.[44] Informal carers are essential in achieving the patient preference of home death.

A further UK study found that 23% of people die at home, presenting two paradoxes: most dying people would prefer to remain at home, but most of them die in institutions; and the majority of the final year is spent at home, but most people are admitted to hospital to die.[45] Indeed, informal carers' inability to cope was a common reason for unplanned admissions, and their needs must be met to achieve policy goals of home-based care as well as increasing government recognition of the importance of carer assessment and support.

The reasons for lack of home deaths are often social and rooted among informal caregivers, rather than medical and relating to the patient. UK government policy in the last decade has recognized the capacities of informal carers, and has attempted to meet their needs via the Carers (Recognition and Services) Act 1995. Department of Health guidance has set standards for quality assurance in services for carers, including the formulation of clearly defined aims and objectives, evaluation, and details of how the aims will be met. This intention of the Act is to enhance existing informal support networks, and to integrate family members into service-based support.

The social exclusion resulting from informal caring carries important social policy implications. How best to support informal carers offers a unique set of challenges in the palliative care context. Defining terminal illness is difficult, because some patients live for long periods with terminal conditions and the trajectory of dying is uncertain. Carers are faced with considerable uncertainty over the length of time they are committing themselves to care, and what may be involved in delivering that care.[46]

The identity of the informal carer in palliative care has been confused and ambiguous, but how we perceive carers is fundamental to their well-being and support.[47] The processes of needs assessment and specific service provision for carers will encourage services to consider how they perceive carers. Although hospice and palliative care services advocate a family-centered care approach, research and care services have often cast the carer in the proxy role, as a provider of information, and therefore as an extension of the patient.[48] However, the carer can be seen as holding a unique position of both providing *and* needing support, and indeed it has been suggested that it is sometimes unclear who is 'the patient'.[49] The service conceptualization of the carer as co-worker rather than client is problematic and leaves unmet support needs.[50] Models of supportive intervention need to carefully consider how they provide for carers, because it may not be appropriate to simply incorporate carers into existing nursing provision.[51]

Although the palliative care model has focused on the family, the identification of carers on behalf of services is more problematic than it may appear.[52] A carer may not be actively giving care, the carer themselves may be receiving nursing care, care may be provided by more than one person, or the carer may not be a family member. Although the policy of community care underpins home palliative care, friends may be disenfranchised or excluded by professionals.[53] Friends and neighbors are a small but considerable resource, and providers of support services need to ensure that they do not overlook this group of carers, who may have needs while also providing valuable community-based support.

The difficulties faced by professionals in identifying carers are compounded by the lack of identification with the label of 'carer' by those providing informal care.[54] Informal carers are often unaware that they fit the definition of a carer, and many are unaware of their rights to assessment or the availability of services.[55] A

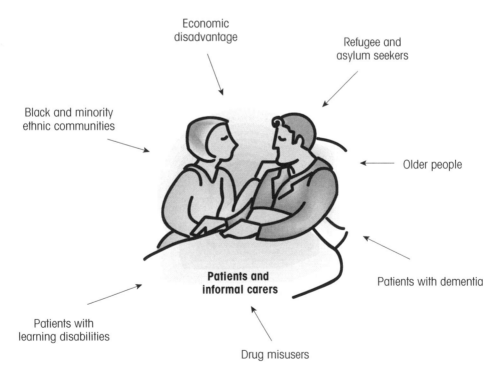

**FIGURE 2.2** Factors that influence access to palliative care provision for patients with advanced disease and their informal carers

significant challenge to professional service attempts to support informal carers is the ambivalence felt by carers towards their role and identity.[56] Carers rarely identify with the label, do not see themselves as credible service recipients, and therefore are reluctant to present their needs, are unwilling to use palliative care service resources that could be allocated to patient care, and tend to cope by not engaging with their needs until the bereavement phase.

There is a significant body of evidence for a high frequency of multi-dimensional unmet needs among informal carers of dependants with advanced disease, which include information, psychological support, nursing and practical care, management of fatigue, and financial assistance.[57] However, how best to meet these many needs is far from clear from the current body of evidence. A systematic review of interventions for carers in cancer and palliative care found that 23 reported interventions, of which nine were targeted services for carers, and only six had been evaluated. The quality of the evidence was generally poor.

Although it is clear that home palliative care is the preferred modality of palliative care for patients and policy makers, the needs of carers are largely unmet and may exceed those of the patient. This carries implications for care breakdown, unplanned admissions, and poor outcomes for carers and patients. However, there is a chronic lack of evidence on how practitioners should best support this population, and a range of evaluated interventions that seek to address each of the primary domains of need is urgently required.


## The economically deprived

Britain leads Western Europe in its poverty, with twice as many poor households as Belgium, Denmark, Italy, Holland or Sweden. A quarter of men of working age were 'non-employed' in 1996, and a quarter of households existed on less than half the national average income, after housing costs, in the early 1990s.[58] While overall personal income rose substantially in the 1980s and 1990s, the gap between the richest and the poorest has grown dramatically.[59]

Evidence from a number of studies suggests that between 50 and 70% of patients would prefer to be cared for at home for as long as possible, and to die at home given the choice.[60] In areas of high socio-economic deprivation, however, fewer people do die at home. They are more likely to die in a hospital and less likely to die in a hospice compared to other groups.[61,62] They also die at younger ages,[63] often with a poorer quality of life.[64] If specialist palliative care services are available in these areas, they tend to require more resources to achieve the same level of care than in areas where deprivation is lower.[65]

Figure 2.3 illustrates the wide variation in deaths at home, by deprivation band.[66] It would appear that lower occupational groups are at a disadvantage, both in terms of home death and in access to cancer-related services.

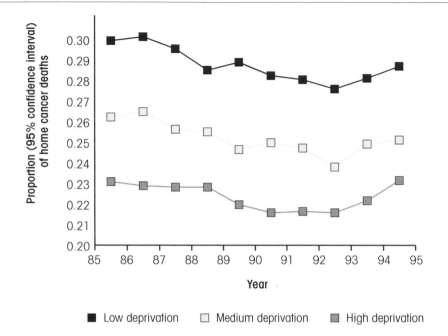

**FIGURE 2.3** Trends in deaths at home from cancer by deprivation band (⅓ population sorted by score of deprivation)

Source: Higginson et al., 1999[∞]

## Older people

The phenomenon of demographic ageing, which refers to the increasing share of the population that is elderly, presents a growing challenge to health and social care services in developed countries. Most people who die are old, and their needs are sometimes complex as a result of multiple morbidities. While fair access lies at the heart of good public services in some areas of health and social care, older people and their carers have experienced age-based discrimination in access to and availability of services.[67] Older people from black and minority ethnic groups can be particularly disadvantaged.[68]

It has long been suggested that the palliative care movement has not afforded older patients adequate care, preferring to devote more of its resources to relatively younger people.[69] While some research has, in part, rebutted this accusation, an analysis of minimum data set activity for hospices and hospital palliative care services in 1997 and 1998 demonstrated that age does represent an important influence in determining which patients receive specialist palliative care.[70]

In general terms, older people are less likely to be cared for at home and more likely to be in nursing and residential homes, where staff are often ill equipped to manage the symptoms associated with advanced disease. In an evaluation of the adequacy of pain management in nursing homes in five states in the USA, Bernabei *et al.* found that pain was prevalent among nursing home residents and was often untreated, particularly among older patients.[71] Similar concerns have been raised in the UK.[72]

## People with dementia

In recent years dementia has become a major concern for all developed countries, and greatly affects the use of primary and secondary health services and social care.[73] People with severe mental illness require a range of skilled professional care with expertise in their management. The focus on their mental health problems can lead to the under-diagnosis of life-threatening illnesses and to the under-recognition and under-treatment of symptoms.

Dementia can legitimately be seen as a terminal illness, and patients die with this mental illness.[74] Further, new variant Creutzfeldt Jakob disease (CJD) may also become a significant cause of dementia in younger people in the future. Recent research has indicated that many patients with dementia have symptoms and health needs comparable to those who have cancer, but for longer periods of time.[75] These results indicate that many patients with dementia have unmet disease-related concerns that, although they can be met by generalist health and social services support, are nevertheless amenable to specialist palliative care.

## People with learning disabilities

In the early 1990s the Department of Health in the UK adopted the term 'learning disability' as the successor to other terms such as 'learning difficulty' (which is still used in relation to the education of children), mental handicap, mental sub-normality, mental retardation (used in the USA), and mental deficiency. 'Learning disability', the term used in this chapter, is preferable because it describes the effect of lower-than-average intelligence in a manner consistent with the WHO definitions of impairment, disability and handicap.[76]

It has been argued that people with learning disabilities are among the most socially excluded and vulnerable groups in the UK today. Very few have jobs, live in their own homes, or have real choice over who cares for them. Producing precise information on the number of people with learning disabilities in the population is difficult, however. The UK government's White Paper, *Valuing People*,[77] suggests that there may be approximately 210 000 people described as having severe and profound learning disabilities, and approximately 1.2 million people with mild or moderate learning disabilities, in England.

Empirical knowledge of the general health needs of people with learning disabilities has increased in recent years. Research indicates that this client group have more demanding health needs than the general population and are also experiencing increased life expectancy, especially among people with Down's syndrome.[78] Increased life expectancy has in part been due to advances in medical treatments that are now available to this group of people. However, this has resulted in the increased incidence of progressive disease, such as myocardial and vascular disease, cancer and Alzheimer's disease.[79] Surveys have increasingly shown that many people with learning disabilities have undetected conditions that cause unnecessary suffering or reduce the quality or length of their lives.[80–82]

Failure to diagnose advanced disease for this population group may mean that not only are treatment options limited but also that the window for accessing palliative care becomes truncated. This prevents both patients and their caregivers from adequately planning and preparing for the final stages of their advanced illness.[83] Once the opportunity for palliative care presents itself, problems continue. Little is known about how people with learning disabilities experience pain, and evidence suggests they many experience difficulties communicating its presence.[84] Other symptoms (e.g. nausea, fatigue or dysphagia) are similarly poorly communicated by individuals or poorly understood by health care professionals, and this may result in their sub-optimal assessment and management.[85,86]

## People from black and minority ethnic groups

Ethnicity is difficult to define, but most definitions reflect self-identification with cultural traditions that provide both a meaningful social identity and boundaries between groups.[87] At the time of writing, people from Black and minority ethnic backgrounds represent approximately 8.1% of the population in the UK. Although there is a significant lack of data about people from minority ethnic communities, the available data from the UK, the USA and Australia confirm that some groups experience disproportionate disadvantage across the board. More often than not they are concentrated in deprived areas and suffer all the problems that affect other people in these areas.[36]

People from minority ethnic communities also suffer the consequences of overt and inadvertent racial discrimination – individual and institutional – and an inadequate recognition and understanding of other complexities they may experience (e.g. barriers such as language, cultural and religious differences). They also experience social invisibility where routinely collected data from a number of sources are either wholly or partially inadequate. Death registration certificates only record country of origin or country of birth, not ethnicity,[88] hospital minimum data set information and cancer registration data frequently omit self-assigned ethnicity, or classifications of ethnic difference are outdated or applied incorrectly.

**BOX 2.3** Black and minority ethnic social exclusion at the end of life: why does it occur?

| | |
|---|---|
| **Social deprivation**<br>Low socio-economic status has been positively linked to an increased likelihood of hospital deaths, although this would apply equally to all population groups.[97] | **Attitudes to palliative care**<br>Barriers to healthcare that the poor and the disenfranchised have traditionally encountered may affect their receptivity to palliative care.[98] |
| **Knowledge of specialist palliative care services and poor communication**<br>There is a growing body of evidence that Black and ethnic minorities are not adequately aware of specialist palliative care services available to them.[99–101] | **Dissatisfaction with health care**<br>Uptake of health and social services among certain minority ethnic communities has revealed lower utilization of services due to dissatisfaction of services.[102]<br><br>**Mistrust**<br>Evidence from the USA supports the contention that Black and minority ethnic groups are less likely than White patients to trust the motivations of doctors who discuss end-of-life care with them.[103] |
| **Ethno-centrism**<br>Demand for services may be influenced by the 'ethnocentric' outlook of palliative care services, discouraging Black and minority ethnic groups from making use of relevant provision.[104] | **Gatekeepers**<br>Some healthcare professionals act as 'gatekeepers' to services among minority ethnic groups, contributing to lower referral rates.[105] |

Although a number of explanations have been advanced to account for the poor uptake of services among Black and minority ethnic groups, few studies have actually quantified the palliative care needs and problems of patients with advanced disease and their carers, in different communities (*see* Box 2.3). Most recently, a study in an inner-London health authority demonstrated that first-generation Black Caribbean patients with advanced disease experienced restricted access to some specialist palliative care services compared to native-born White UK deceased patients,[89,90] yet an analysis of local provision revealed no lack of palliative care services.[91] This example of under-utilization of palliative care services by the Black Caribbean community at the end of life supports other research among minority ethnic communities in the UK, Australia and the USA.[92-96]

## Refugees and asylum seekers

Estimating the total number of refugees and asylum seekers worldwide is difficult, because definitions differ widely. In the UK, refugees are defined as those who have been granted indefinite leave to remain or have permanent residence. Asylum seekers are those who have submitted an application for protection under the Geneva Convention and are waiting for the claim to be decided by the Home Office. At the time of writing there are around 230 000 people in this category living in the UK and numbers continue to increase.[106] Refugees and asylum seekers form significant minority populations in many UK towns and cities. It is extremely difficult to obtain demographic information on these groups at the local level, and this lack of information represents one of the difficulties in developing accessible services for them.[107]

Although refugees and asylum seekers are often grouped together, they are not necessarily a homogeneous group, and have varying experiences and needs.[108] Many refugees have health problems, such as parasitic or nutritional diseases,[109] and diseases such as hepatitis, tuberculosis and HIV and AIDS, which frequently overlap with problems of social deprivation. Their health problems are also amplified by family separation, hostility and racism from the host population, poverty and social isolation.[109-111]

Individuals from sub-Saharan Africa, many of whom may be refugees and asylum seekers, make up the second-largest group of people affected by HIV in the UK.[112] They are more likely to be socially disadvantaged and isolated, to be much less aware of the healthcare to which they are entitled, and to be more likely to present only when symptomatic. Experience has shown that this patient group continues to require palliative care despite the advances made with highly active antiretroviral therapy (HAART), because they tend to present late with AIDS-related illnesses and have higher rates of tuberculosis, both of which are linked to a poorer prognosis. For many patients who do not have a GP and are reluctant to register with one, lack of a stable home environment and reluctance to access local services may mean that dying at home is not an option.[113]

## Drug users

In England, during the year 2000–01, the number of drug misusers reported as receiving treatment from both drug misuse agencies and GPs was approximately 118 500.[114] There is very little literature on how drug misusers utilize specialist palliative care services. The meager literature that does exist focuses mainly on issues of pain control for this population. A single exploratory study in the USA explored the experiences of hospices providing care to intravenous HIV/AIDs drug users.[115] The survey revealed that the provision of community palliative care for these patients was frequently problematic because of patients' poor living conditions, many of which were considered unsafe to visit. Other challenges included healthcare professionals' concerns that patients might be resistant to hospice care if they perceived the hospice as a barrier to their continued drug use.

It has been suggested that drug users require a modified healthcare system, which understands and considers the problems of drug users, but that the initiation and maintenance of contact may require a variety of initiatives.[116] Morrison and Ruben[117] similarly argue that services need to deliver care to these groups in imaginative and innovative ways that are not judgmental and encourage contact without reinforcing traditional stereotypes. Without appropriate services, they argue, high levels of mortality among drug users will continue.

## Prisoners

In 2005 there were an estimated 76 017 prisoners in England and Wales, of whom 5792 were serving life sentences.[118] Historically, prison healthcare has been organized outside the NHS. This has given rise to questions about equity, standards, professional isolation and whether the Prison Service has the capacity to carry out its healthcare function.[119] The Government is now committed to developing a range of proposals aimed at improving healthcare for prisoners. The aims include ensuring prisoners have access to the same quality and range of healthcare services as the general public receives from the NHS by promoting a closer partnership between the NHS and the Prison Service at local, regional and national levels.

Very little UK literature has focused on the palliative care needs of prisoners, and that available is largely descriptive or relates to single case histories.[120,121] More research has taken place in the USA, where a number of palliative care programs have been developed for prisoners (e.g. the Louisiana State Penitentiary at Angola.[122] This has been largely because in Louisiana the sentencing laws are tougher than any other state in the USA, the courts hand out a disproportionate number of life sentences, and few of these prisoners are granted parole. As a result, an estimated 85% of Angola's 5200 inmates will grow old and die there.[122]

There are a number of problems in introducing palliative care into prisons, not least the mutual distrust between staff and prisoners. Effective symptom control, particularly adequate pain control, can be difficult under these circumstances. Drugs to manage pain control may be used for other illicit purposes. Also, visiting from family and friends can be restricted, not least because the prison may be located at some distance from family.

## The magnitude of the problem: implications for palliative care policy and service development

Since the introduction of the NHS in the UK, and in other countries where social welfare has become commonplace, health care has been more widely extended to many sections of the population. However, universal access to care and treatment has remained elusive. Palliative care provided by the modern hospice movement, with laudable aspirations to extend the right to care as widely as possible, has been shown to be inequitable on a number of fronts. This chapter has revealed that silent sections of the population are ignored or inadequately served at the end of life. Solutions to the problems come in many forms, none of which will be successful in isolation.

First, health and social care professionals' knowledge and attitudes about engaging socially excluded populations must be improved.[123] This concern can be addressed, in part, through a comprehensive needs assessment, be it epidemiological (including a deeper understanding of demographic and economic factors that impact on the experience of advanced disease and providing informal care), comparative or corporate, including the meaningful collation and interpretation of experiences and views from a variety of sources. These include the views of patients and informal carers, providers of care, as well as purchasers and planners.

A number of regional implementation groups which have successfully undertaken similar exercises in order to plan palliative care services in their own areas offer the potential to explore strategies at an epidemiological and corporate level (e.g. in London[124] and Wales[125]). Both established a framework for the development of local policies and recommended closer links between agencies involved in the provision of care. Significantly, they have recommended devoting more resources to research that explores the unmet palliative care needs of the socially excluded, given the paucity of evidence in certain areas. Without more comprehensive information, moving these complex agendas forward remains a challenge.

Second, there is an urgent need to raise public awareness of palliative care services and to provide public education about the care provided to reduce any misconceptions about services that may be influencing access. Information provided to NHS Direct and Primary Care Trusts (PCTs) may also be important.

Lastly, the charitable sector is uniquely suited to support new ideas that extend care to the point where it can be integrated into society and become the social norm rather than the exception. Despite differences in the funding arrangements of care in the USA, the Robert Wood Johnson Foundation and the Health Resources and Services Administration (HRSA) have been successful in pump-priming pilot projects to increase access to palliative care to socially deprived communities[126,127] (*see* Box 2.4). In recent years the UK has followed suit (*see* Box 2.5). Although palliative care cannot completely remove the impact of the advanced disease, approaches must be sought to extend its lessons to all those who stand to benefit from its increasing sophistication.

**BOX 2.4** Example of a US public sector-sponsored venture to care for HIV/AIDS palliative care patients

> A Special Projects for National Significance initiative of the HIV/AIDS Bureau of the Health Resources and Services Administration (HRSA) has recently been set up to provide funds for palliative care services in Alabama, Baltimore and New York for individuals with advanced disease who have difficulty accessing healthcare systems.

**BOX 2.5** Example of UK charitable sector-sponsored venture to manage underserved patients with advanced cancer and their informal carers

> A 'Palliative Care Pathway', funded through the New Opportunities Fund, has recently been developed in North West London, focusing specifically on previously 'hard-to-access' socially excluded patients with advanced cancer and their families. The aim of the project is to develop referral criteria, an interdisciplinary core assessment tool, and associated documentation for use by health and social care professionals to improve end-of-life decisions for pathway patients and their caregivers.

Although palliative care cannot completely remove the impact of progressive disease, comprehensive rigorous needs assessments must be conducted and innovative approaches sought to extend palliative care to all those who stand to benefit from its increasing sophistication. A summary of questions to explore is presented in Box 2.6.

**BOX 2.6** Summary of questions to ask when planning a palliative care needs assessment

- What is your area of interest? (This defines the scope of palliative care needs to be addressed.)
- Are you interested in a whole population or a particular sub-section (for example, older people or Black and minority ethnic groups)?
- What is the exact size of the problem? How many people share that palliative care need?
- What are the views of patients with advanced disease, their informal carers, and the local community? What is known from previous work?
- Who else do you need to talk to locally (e.g. family doctors, community nurses, palliative care physicians and clinical nurse specialists, social workers, chaplains etc.)?
- How do your figures compare with local and national averages? How important is the problem in your locality compared with others?
- What interventions are you already making? Do you have a response to the problem?
- What are other agencies doing?
- What has worked elsewhere? Is there any relevant literature available or projects that can be visited? Are there examples of 'best practice' in the area you are interested in?
- What could and should you be doing in future? Consider all options, prioritize, and develop an action plan.

Adapted from: Sheffield Health Authority. *A 'Toolkit' for Health Needs Assessment in Primary Care* (LAPIS). Sheffield: Sheffield Health; 1996.

## References

1  Hinton J. *Dying.* London: Penguin; 1967.
2  Higginson IJ. Health care needs assessment: palliative and terminal care. In: Stevens A, Raftery J, editors. *Health Care Needs Assessment.* Oxford: Radcliffe Medical Press; 1997: 183–260.
3  Ingelton C, Skilbeck J, Clark D. Needs assessment for palliative care: three projects compared. *Palliat Med.* 2004; **15**: 398–404.
4  WHO Expert Committee. *Cancer Pain Relief and Palliative Care.* World Health Organization Technical Report Series No. 804. Geneva: World Health Organization; 1990.
5  World Health Organization. *Report on Five Countries: palliative care in emerging Sub Saharan Africa.* Geneva: WHO; 2002.

6  Addington-Hall J, Higginson IJ. *Palliative Care for Non-cancer Patients.* Oxford: Oxford University Press; 2001.

7  Soper K. *On Human Needs.* Sussex: Harvester Press; 1981.

8  Bradshaw J. The taxonomy of social need. In: McLachlan G, editor. *Problems and Progress in Medical Care: essays on current research.* Oxford: Oxford University Press; 1972: 71–82.

9  Higginson IJ, Goodwin DM. Needs assessment in day care. In: Hearn J, Myers K, editors. *Palliative Day Care in Practice.* Oxford: Oxford University Press; 2001: 12–22.

10  Stevens A, Raftery J. Introduction. In: Stevens A, Raftery J, editors. *Health Care Needs Assessment: the epidemiologically based needs assessment reviews, Vol 1.* Oxford: Radcliffe Medical Press; 1994.

11  Franks PJ. Need for palliative care. In: Bosanquet N, Salisbury C, editors. *Providing a Palliative Care Service: towards an evidence base.* Oxford: Oxford University Press; 1999: 43–56.

12  Higginson IJ. Palliative and terminal care. In: Stevens A, Raftery J, editors. *Health Care Needs Assessment: the epidemiologically based needs assessment reviews.* Oxford: Radcliffe Medical Press; 1997.

13  Cartwright A. Changes in life and care in the year before death 1969–1987. *J Pub Health Med.* 1991; **13**: 81–7.

14  Seale C. A comparison of hospice and conventional care. *Soc Sci Med.* 1991; **32**: 147–52.

15  Field D, Douglas C, Jagger C, *et al.* Terminal illness: views of patients and their lay carers. *Palliat Med.* 1995; **9**: 45–54.

16  Bennett M, Corcoran G. The impact on community palliative care services of a hospital palliative care team. *Palliat Med.* 1994; **8**: 237–44.

17  Higginson IJ, Wade AM, McCarthy M. Effectiveness of two palliative support teams. *J Pub Health Med.* 1992; **14**: 50–6.

18  Addington-Hall JM, MacDonald L, Anderson H, *et al.* Dying from cancer: the views of bereaved family and friends about the experiences of terminally ill patients. *Palliat Med.* 1991; **5**: 207–14.

19  McPherson CJ, Addington-Hall JM. Judging the quality of care at the end of life: can proxies provide reliable information? *Soc Sci Med.* 2003; **56**: 95–109.

20  Addington-Hall JM, McCarthy M. Regional study of care for the dying: methods and sample characteristics. *Palliat Med.* 1995; **9**: 27–35.

21  Addington-Hall J, McCarthy M. Dying of cancer: results of a national population-based investigation. *Palliat Med.* 1995; **9**: 295–305.

22  Frankel S, Kammerling M. Assessing the need for hospice beds. *Health Trends.* 1990; 22: 83–86.

23  Eve A, Jackson A. Palliative care, where are we now? *Palliat Care Today.* 1994; 22–3.

24  Murtagh FEM, Preston M, Higginson IJ. Patterns of dying: palliative care for non-malignant disease. *Clin Med.* 2004; 4(1): 39–44.

25  Hockley JM, Dunlop R, Davies RJ. Survey of distressing symptoms in dying patients and their families in hospital and the response to a symptom control team. *BMJ* 1988; **296**: 1715–17.

26  Severs MP, Wilkins PSW. A hospital palliative care ward for elderly people. *Age Ageing.* 1991; **20**: 361–4.

27  Noble B. *A Snapshot Survey of Hospital and Hospice Patients: older peoples: palliative*

*care strategy.* Appendix B. Sheffield: Health Authority and Family Health Services Authority; 1993.

28  Mor V, McHorney C, Sherwood S. Secondary morbidity among the recently bereaved. *Am J Psychiatry.* 1986; **143**(2): 158–62.

29  Norris FH, Murrell SA. Older adult family stress and adaptation before and after bereavement. *J Gerontol.* 1987; **42**: 606–12.

30  Wiles R, Payne S, Jarret N. Improving palliative care services: a pragmatic model for evaluating services and assessing unmet need. *Palliat Med.* 1999; **13**: 131–7.

31  Clark D, Malson H. Key issues in palliative care needs assessment. *Prog Palliat Care.* 1995; **3**: 53–5.

32  Hart JT. The inverse care law. *Lancet* 1971; **1**: 405–12.

33  Goddard M, Smith P. Equity of access to health care services: theory and evidence from the UK. *Soc Sci Med.* 2001; **53**: 1149–62.

34  Townsend P, Davison N. *Inequalities in Health: the Black Report.* Harmondsworth: Penguin; 1982.

35  Whitehead M. *Inequalities in Health: the Black Report and the health divide.* Harmondsworth: Penguin; 1992.

36  Department of Health. *Inequalities in Health: report of an independent inquiry chaired by Sir Donald Acheson.* London: The Stationery Office; 1998.

37  Addington-Hall JM. *Positive Partnerships: palliative care for adults with severe mental health problems.* London: National Council for Hospices and Specialist Palliative Care Services; 2000.

38  O'Neill J, Marconi K. Access to palliative care in the USA: why emphasize vulnerable populations? *J R Soc Med.* 2001; **94**: 452–4.

39  Seymour J, Clark D, Marples R. Palliative care and policy in England: a review of health improvement plans for 1999–2003. *Palliat Med.* 2002; **16**(1): 5–11.

40  Higginson IJ, Goodwin DM. Needs assessment in day care. In: Hearn J, Myers K, editors. *Palliative Day Care in Practice.* Oxford: Oxford University Press; 2001: 12–22.

41  Barratt H. The health of the excluded. *BMJ* 2001; **323**: 240.

42  Social Exclusion Unit. *Preventing Social Exclusion.* London: The Stationery Office; 2001.

43  Koffman J, Snow P. Carers of dependants with advanced disease. In: Addington-Hall J, Higginson IJ, editors. *Palliative Care for Non-Cancer Patients.* Oxford: Oxford University Press; 2001: 227–38.

44  Schulz R, Beach S. Caregiving as a risk factor for mortality. *JAMA* 1999; **282**: 2215–19.

45  Thorpe G. Enabling more dying people to die at home. *BMJ* 1993; **307**: 915–18.

46  Payne S, Ellis-Hill C. *The Future: interventions and conceptual issues: chronic and terminal illness: new perspectives on caring and carers.* Oxford: Oxford University Press; 2001.

47  Lobchuck MM, Kristjanson L, Degner L, *et al.* Perceptions of symptom distress in lung cancer patients. I: congruence between patients and primary family caregivers. *J Pain Sympt Manage.* 1997; **14**: 136–46.

48  Neale B, Clark D. Informal care of people with cancer: a review of research on needs and services. *J Cancer Care.* 1992; **1**: 193–8.

49  Northouse LL, Peters-Golden H. Cancer and the family: strategies to assist spouses. *Sem in Oncol Nurs.* 1993; **9**: 74–82.

50  Payne S, Smith P, Dean S. Identifying the concerns of informal carers in palliative care. *Palliat Med.* 1999; **13**: 37–44.

51 Ferrell BR, Grant M, Chan J, *et al.* The impact of cancer pain education on family caregivers of elderly patients. *Oncol Nurs Forum.* 1995; **22**: 1211–18.

52 Higginson IJ. Defining the unit of care: who are we supporting and how? In: Bruera E, Portenay R, editors. *Topics in Palliative Care.* Oxford: Oxford University Press; 1998: 205–7.

53 Young E, Seale C, Bury M. It's not like family going is it?: negotiating friendship boundaries towards the end of life. *Mortality.* 1998; **3**: 27–42.

54 Hunt M. The identification and provision of care for the terminally ill at home by 'family' members. *Sociol Health Ill.* 1991; **13**: 375–95.

55 Henwood M. Helping the helpers. *Community Care.* 1998; 22–4.

56 Harding R, Higginson IJ. Working with ambivalence: informal carers of patients at the end of life. *Support Cancer Care.* 2001; **9**: 642–5.

57 Higginson IJ, Wade A, McCarthy M. Palliative care: views of patients and their families. *BMJ* 1990; **301**: 277–81.

58 Walker E, Walker C. *Britain Divided: the growth of social exclusion in the 1980s and 1990s.* London: Child Poverty Action Group; 1997.

59 Office for National Statistics. *Social Trends.* London: The Stationery Office; 2000.

60 Gomes B, Higginson IJ. Home or hospital: choices at the end of life. *J R Soc Med.* 2004; **97**: 413–14.

61 Higginson IJ, Webb D, Lessof L. Reducing hospital beds for patients with advanced cancer. *Lancet* 1994; **344**: 409.

62 Sims A, Radford J, Doran K, *et al.* Social class variation in place of death. *Palliat Med.* 1997; **11**: 369–73.

63 Soni Raleigh V, Kiri A. Life expectancy in England: variations and trends by gender, health authority and level of deprivation. *J Epidem Comm Health.* 1997; **51**: 649–58.

64 Cartwright A. Social class differences in health and care in the year before death. *J Epidem Comm Health.* 1992; **46**: 54–7.

65 Clark C. Social deprivation increases workload in palliative care of terminally ill patients. *BMJ* 1997; **314**: 1202.

66 Higginson IJ, Jarman B, Astin P, *et al.* Do social factors affect where patients die: an analysis of 10 years of cancer deaths in England. *J Pub Health Med.* 1999; **21**: 22–8.

67 Age Concern. *Turning Your Back on Us: older people and the NHS.* London: Age Concern; 1999.

68 Department of Health. *They Look After Their Own, Don't They?* CI(98)2. London: Department of Health; 1998.

69 Seymour J, Clark D, Philp I. Palliative care and geriatric medicine: shared concerns, shared challenges. *Palliat Med.* 2001; **15**: 269–70.

70 Eve A, Higginson IJ. Minimum dataset activity for hospice and hospital palliative care services in the UK 1997/98. *Palliat Med.* 2000; **14**: 395–404.

71 Bernabei R, Gambassi G, Lapane K, *et al.* Management of pain in elderly patients with cancer. [erratum in *JAMA* 1999; **281**(2): 136]. *JAMA* 1998; **279**: 1877–82.

72 Komaromy C, Sidell M, Katz J. Dying in care: factors which influence the quality of terminal care given to older people in residential and nursing homes. *Int J Palliat Nurs* 2000; **6**: 192–205.

73 Koffman J, Fulop NJ, Pashley D, *et al.* No way out: the use of elderly mentally ill acute and assessment psychiatric beds in north and south Thames regions. *Age Ageing.* 1996; **25**: 268–72.

74  Addington-Hall J. *Positive Partnerships: palliative care for adults with severe mental health problems.* London: National Council for Hospices and Specialist Palliative Care Services; 2000.

75  McCarthy M, Addington-Hall JM, Altmann D. The experience of dying with dementia: a retrospective survey. *Int J Geriatr Psychiatry.* 1997; **12**: 404–9.

76  World Health Organization. *International Classification of Impairments, Disabilities, and Handicaps: a manual relating to the consequences of diseases.* Geneva: World Health Organization; 1980.

77  Secretary of State for Health. *Valuing People: a new strategy for learning disability for the 21st century.* CM 5086. London: The Stationery Office; 2001.

78  NHS Executive. *Signpost for Successful Commissioning and Providing Health Services for People with Learning Difficulties.* London: The Stationery Office; 1998.

79  Jancar J. Consequences of a longer life for the mentally handicapped. *Am J Ment Retard.* 1993; **98**: 285–92.

80  Tuffrey-Wijne I. Care of the terminally ill. *Learn Disabil Pract.* 1998; **1**: 8–11.

81  Howells G. Are the medical needs of mentally handicapped adults being met? *Br J Gen Pract.* 1986; **36**: 453.

82  Keenan P, McIntosh P. Learning disabilities and palliative care. *Palliat Care Today.* 2000; 11–13.

83  Brown H. The service needs of people with learning disabilities who are dying. *Psychol Res.* 2000; **10**: 39–47.

84  Beirsdorff K. Pain intensity and indifference: alternative explanations for some medical catastrophes. *Ment Retard.* 1991; **29**: 359–62.

85  Tuffrey-Wijne I. Palliative care and learning disabilities. *Nurs Times.* 1997; **93**: 50–1.

86  Tuffrey-Wijne I. Care of the terminally ill. *Learning Disability Pract.* 1998; **1**: 8–11.

87  Senior A, Bhopal R. Ethnicity as a variable in epidemiological research. *BMJ* 1994; **309**: 327–30.

88  Koffman J, Higginson IJ. Minority ethnic groups and *Our Healthier Nation. J Pub Health Med.* 2000; 22(2): 245.

89  Koffman J, Higginson IJ. Accounts of satisfaction with health care at the end of life: a comparison of first generation black Caribbeans and white patients with advanced disease. *Palliat Med.* 2001; **15**: 337–45.

90  Koffman J, Higginson IJ. Dying to be home? A comparison of preferred place of death of first generation black Caribbean and native-born white patients in the United Kingdom. *J Palliat Med.* 2004; **7**: 628–36.

91  Eve A, Smith AM, Tebbit P. Hospice and palliative care in the UK 1994–5, including a summary of trends 1990–5. *Palliat Med.* 1997; **11**: 31–43.

92  Farrell J. *Do Disadvantaged and Minority Ethnic Groups Receive Adequate Access to Palliative Care Services?* Glasgow University; 2000.

93  Skilbeck J, Corner J, Beech N, *et al.* Clinical nurse specialists in palliative care. Part 1: a description of the Macmillan Nurse caseload. *Palliat Med.* 2002; **16**: 285–96.

94  Iwashyna TJ, Chang VW. Racial and ethnic differences in place of death: United States, 1993. *J Am Geriatric Soc.* 2002; **50**: 1113–17.

95  Weitzen S, Teno J, Fennel M, *et al.* Factors associated with site of death: a national study of where people die. *Med Care.* 2003; **41**: 323–35.

96  Prior D. Palliative care in marginalised communities. *Prog Palliat Care.* 1999; **7**: 109–15.

97 Higginson IJ, Webb D, Lessof L. Reducing hospital beds for patients with advanced cancer. *Lancet* 1994; **344**: 409.

98 Gibson R. Palliative care for the poor and disenfranchised: a view from the Robert Wood Johnson Foundation. *J R Soc Med.* 2001; **94**: 486–9.

99 Harron-Iqbal H, Field D, Parker H, *et al.* Palliative care services in Leicester. *Int J Palliat Nurs.* 1995; **1**: 114–16.

100 Smaje C, Field D. Absent minorities?: ethnicity and the use of palliative care services. In: Hockey J, Small N, editors. *Death, Gender and Ethnicity.* London: Routledge; 1997: 142–65.

101 Kurent JE, DesHarnais S, Jones W, *et al.* End-of-life decision making for patients with end-stage CHF and terminal malignancies: impact of ethnic and cultural variables. *J Palliat Med.* 2002; **5**: 1999.

102 Lindsay J, Jagger C, Hibbert M, *et al.* Knowledge, uptake and the availability of health and social services among Asian Gujarati and white persons. *Ethn Health.* 1997; **2**: 59–69.

103 Caralis PV, Davis B, Wright K, *et al.* The influence of ethnicity and race on attitudes toward advanced directives, life-prolonging treatments, and euthanasia. *J Clin Ethics.* 1993; **4**: 155–65.

104 Smaje C, Field D. Absent minorities?: ethnicity and the use of palliative care services. In: Hockey J, Small N, editors. *Death, Gender and Ethnicity.* London: Routledge; 1997: 142–65.

105 Cartwright A. Changes in life and care in the year before death 1969–1987. *J Pub Health Med.* 1991; **13**: 81–7.

106 Burnett A, Peel M. What brings asylum seekers to the United Kingdom? *BMJ* 2001; **322**: 485–8.

107 Bardsley M, Hamm J, Lowdell C, *et al. Developing Health Assessment for Black and Minority Ethnic Groups: analysing routine health information.* London: Health of Londoners Project; 2000.

108 Burnett A, Fassil Y. *Meeting the Health Needs of Refugees and Asylum Seekers in the UK: an information and resource pack for health workers.* London: Department of Health; 2002.

109 Jones D, Gill PS. Refugees and primary care: tackling the inequalities. *BMJ* 1998; **317**: 1444–6.

110 Bardsley M, Storkey M. Estimating the numbers of refugees in London. *J Public Health Med.* 2000; **22**: 406–12.

111 Kisely S, Stevens M, Hart B, *et al.* Health issues of asylum seekers and refugees. *Aust NZ J Pub Health.* 2002; **26**: 8–10.

112 Brogan G, George R. HIV/AIDS: symptoms and the impact of new treatments. *Palliat Med.* 1999; **1**: 104–10.

113 Easterbrook P, Meadway J. The changing epidemiology of HIV infection: new challenges for HIV palliative care. *J R Soc Med.* 2001; **94**: 448.

114 Department of Health. *Statistical Press Release: statistics from the regional drug misuse databases on drug misusers in treatment in England, 2000/01.* London: Department of Health; 2001.

115 Cox C. Hospice care for injection drug using AIDS patients. *Hospice J.* 1999; **14**: 13–24.

116 Brettle RP. Injection drug use-related HIV infection. In: Adler MW, editor. *ABC of AIDS.* London: BMJ Publishing; 2001.

117 Morrison CL, Ruben SM. The development of healthcare services for drug misusers and prostitutes. *Postgrad Med J.* 1995; **71**: 593–7.

118 National Offender Management Service. *Prison Population and Accommodation Briefing May 2005.* London: NOMS; 2005.

119 Joint Prison Service and National Health Service Executive Working Group. *The Future Organisation of Prison Health Care.* London: Department of Health; 1999.

120 Wilford T. Developing effective palliative care within a prison setting. *Int J Palliat Nurs.* 2001; **7**: 528–30.

121 Oliver D, Cook L. The specialist palliative care of prisoners. *Eur J Palliat Care.* 1998; **5**: 70–80.

122 Project for Dying in America. Dying in prison: a growing problem emerges from behind bars. *PDIA Newsletter.* 1998; **3**: 1–3.

123 O'Neill J, Marconi K. Access to palliative care in the USA: why emphasize vulnerable populations? *J R Soc Med.* 2001; **94**: 452–4.

124 Higginson IJ. *The Palliative Care for Londoners: needs, experience, outcomes and future strategy.* London: London Regional Strategy Group for Palliative Care; 2001.

125 Welsh Office. *Palliative Care in Wales: towards evidence based purchasing.* Cardiff: Welsh Office; 1996.

126 Gibson R. Palliative care for the poor and disenfranchised: a view from the Robert Wood Johnson Foundation. *J R Soc Med.* 2001; **94**: 486–9.

127 Karus DG, Raveis VH, Marconi K, *et al.* Mental health status of clients from three HIV/AIDS palliative care projects. *Palliat Support Care.* 2004; **2**: 125–38.

# CHAPTER 3

# Pathophysiology of life-limiting illnesses

*DAVID CURROW, AMY ABERNETHY*

## Introduction

Palliative care involves the care of patients who arrive at the end of life from a myriad of illnesses, so a comprehensive review of all the possible symptoms and their pathophysiology is beyond the scope of this book. In this chapter, Currow and Abernethy have concentrated on the final weeks of life.

The first part of the chapter concentrates on the systemic effects of life-limiting illness. Regardless of the illness that led to the patient approaching the end of their life, the presentations tend to merge into a 'final common pathway', as multiple organ systems begin to fail. They then discuss comorbid illnesses, which frequently superimpose other symptoms onto the final pathway, and review the most common symptoms that present. Finally, they translate the scientific detail they have presented into lay language in the form of answers to frequently asked questions.

More detail of the presentation and assessment of common presenting symptoms can be found in Chapter 6, and readers interested in studying the pathophysiology, presentation and management of specific symptoms should read these chapters in parallel. For more comprehensive discussions of the pathophysiology of individual symptoms a range of texts is available. A list of some of these is presented at the end of this chapter.

# Systemic effects of life-limiting illnesses

## Clinical manifestations

For most people with a life-limiting illness, disease progression is marked by deterioration in systemic indices – energy, weight and appetite. Assuming there are no other contributing factors that can be modified, rate of progression is an important marker of overall prognosis.

The systemic nature of advanced life-limiting illnesses is surprisingly reproducible across many diseases, leading to what is often referred to as a 'final common pathway'. What starts as an adaptive process to deal with a sustained insult becomes a detrimental cascade of changes ultimately leading to death.[1] This pathway is best characterized as a catabolic state which can only be modified substantially by influencing the underlying pathological life-limiting processes.

Catabolism in this setting affects major metabolic pathways and is considered as a cytokine-mediated progressive process. Changes in inflammatory markers reflect the impact of cytokines on the process. These processes are not limited to end-stage malignancy. There is evidence of this catabolic pathway in people with AIDS, cardiac failure, chronic respiratory diseases, senescence and chronic inflammatory diseases.[2–6]

### Lean body mass

Whatever the life-limiting illness, lean body mass is almost always lost as the disease progresses in a relatively linear fashion for much of the illness's course.[7] This is sometimes attributed to disuse atrophy, and although it can contribute to loss of muscle, disuse is not in itself a complete explanation. Disuse atrophy starts almost immediately in healthy volunteers who have been put to bed. The accelerated loss of lean body mass even in people who are still active despite their life-limiting illness strongly suggests that there is more to the process than disuse alone.

Increased basal rates of gluconeogenesis occur in the setting of uncontrolled malignancy. Tumors largely rely on glucose for energy, which is eventually generated from skeletal muscle amino acids.[8] Mediation of this process is probably due to the role of host- and tumor-generated interleukin-6 (IL-6) and tumor-derived tumor necrosis factor alpha (TNF). The rate of gluconeogenesis is also substantially affected by total tumor mass.[9,10] (By contrast, where cachexia is characterized by protein and fat loss, starvation largely generates fat loss.)[11]

In cancer or AIDS, loss of lean body mass is obvious and in many people's minds characterizes evidence of disease progression. This is both a community perception and the perception of patients with the advanced disease. Of note, people with end-stage organ failure tend to lose lean body mass and, contrary to earlier beliefs, losing lean body mass is not simply due to poor food intake.[12]

In cardiac failure, loss of lean body mass may be masked by generalized oedema. Bioimpedance studies demonstrate the changing characteristics of body composition across time in the setting of life-limiting illnesses, including the extensive loss of muscle.[13]

### Appetite

Appetite is often affected as a life-limiting illness progresses, and in comparison to healthy states, reversing appetite loss does little to reverse loss of lean body mass unless the underlying cause is addressed. Loss of appetite does contribute to inadequate caloric and protein intake, however, especially early in the course of the illness.[7] Changes in appetite may be worsened by changes in taste, but a primary problem remains a decrease in the desire for food.[12]

Specific food preferences can also change as a life-limiting illness progresses. Foods that have been a favourite may not be tolerated. The time of the day when food is sought may also change. For example, specific losses may include the taste for alcohol or red meat.[12]

Food has many connotations: social (it is the time when we most often stop, sit and talk to the people who are close to us in life), well-being ('if you don't eat, you die'), nutritional (concepts of a balanced diet), along with cultural determinants ('good' and 'bad' foods).[14] Relatives will often suggest that people with a life-limiting illness are 'giving up' as food intake wanes.

Total parenteral nutrition is an intuitive response to anorexia and weight loss in life-limiting illness. However, its use has not improved survival rates in spite of advances in antibiotics reducing the morbidity from the serious central venous line infections that may have worsened previous reported outcomes.[15] End-stage loss of appetite is a response to systemic changes from the life-limiting illness, not the driving mechanism of poor nutrition. Providing nutritional substrates in advanced disease does not reverse the underlying catabolic state, and, clearly, the relationship between glucose, fat and protein metabolism in a body systemically affected by cancer is complex.[8]

### Energy

People with life-limiting illnesses describe overwhelming fatigue. Hypermetabolism, secondary to the inflammatory state, may be a factor that partially contributes to this process.[7,11] The fatigue is not reversed by more rest. Indeed, people may say they are just as exhausted after 14 hours' sleep as when they went to bed. This exhaustion, especially late in the course of the illness, progresses in line with the overall systemic progress of the disease. It parallels functional status for many people and allows prognostication by assessing the rate of change in fatigue. If functional status and fatigue are worsening on a monthly basis, prognosis is probably measured in months; if it is worsening objectively on a weekly basis with no other reversible cause, prognosis may well be measured in weeks.

The nexus between caloric intake, lean body mass and energy levels is progressively lost as a catabolic state progresses. In health, we accept a close relationship between these three factors. As any 'expected' death approaches, any relationship between these three factors becomes more tenuous.

## Laboratory data

### Mediators of inflammation

The 'cytokine cascade' helps to maintain the state of health when we are well. It is part of any acute phase reaction to insult – infection, inflammation or other systemic stressors. In a bid to maintain homeostasis, the cytokine cascade responds to insult with a closely regulated feedback loop in health. By contrast, if the insult is too great, the feedback loops fail and homeostatic measures become destructive. There are data that both host and tumor-driven cytokines and prostaglandins have a role to play in the cachexia syndrome of life-limiting illnesses. Animal experiments involving gene knockout models and specific cytokine antibodies demonstrate partial reversal of cachexia syndromes supporting these theories.[9]

In acute viral infections, for example, levels of cytokines rise. Inflammatory markers such as the erythrocyte sedimentation rate (ESR) or C reactive protein (CRP) rise simultaneously. As the insult is contained, levels of cytokines return to background levels and inflammatory markers fall.

Consider the last time you had a significant viral infection. Appetite was diminished, weight was lost and energy stocks were low. A weight loss of a few kilograms, often over a couple of days, is not achieved in health with absolute starvation in the same time period. Other factors are clearly influencing key bodily functions. As the virus is eradicated, the cytokine response declines and a new state of health is achieved.

In advanced life-limiting illness, cytokines such as TNF, interleukin-1, IL-6, and gamma interferon have extensive cellular impacts that explain some of the effects of unregulated secretion in the setting of an overwhelming insult to homeostasis.[11,16,17] At a cellular level, key functions are irrevocably changed. The circulating levels of cytokines remain high, and unlike an infection, eventual down-regulation does not occur.

Systemic changes of cachexia may also be mediated in part by peptides generated by matrix metalloproteinases, which are still being characterized.[10] This includes proteolysis-inducing factor (PIF), which, as a tumor-specific factor, may contribute to the cachexia syndrome.[7] In cardiac cachexia, there is emerging interest in growth hormone and insulin resistance as factors intrinsically bound up in the inflammatory changes leading to cachexia.[18]

### Apoptosis (programmed cell death)

Every cell having a 'use-by date' is a relatively recent concept. The mechanisms that govern such a complex process are still being elucidated. The understanding that apoptosis can be influenced by systemic factors such as cytokines partly explains the systemic failure of a person's body when it is struggling to regain homeostasis at the end of life. Accelerating the process of apoptosis is one role that high levels of cytokines appear to play in end-stage disease – cancer, AIDS, overwhelming sepsis, end-stage organ failure and neurodegenerative diseases.

Senescent disease clearly has apoptosis as one of its key mechanisms. The process of apoptosis in life-limiting illness from neoplastic disease or end-stage organ failure such as cardiac failure is less clear but relates to a number of factors.[19] Although apoptosis may be brought forward in time through systemic neurohumoral mechanisms, it appears not to be the main factor initiating muscle wasting in cachexia. As cachexia progresses in cardiac failure, muscle cell wasting worsens, exercise tolerance deteriorates and fibrosis replaces myocytes in the affected muscles.[20]

## What can be reversed help?

### Exercise

There are emerging data to support exercise as a mediator of systemic changes in a life-limiting illness early in the course of the disease. The data, derived in a range of clinical settings, would support the benefits of tailored exercise programs for people with good levels of function. In late-stage disease, the benefits are not seen and may indeed exacerbate feelings of lethargy and fatigue.

### Nutrition

Nutritional supplements are a focus of much research and even more opinion, especially in the public at large. Every person losing lean body mass with a life-limiting illness is given copious advice by all their family, friends and associates about what they should and should not eat.

There is little evidence of benefit from particular diets. There has been recent interest in the role of eicosapentaenoic acid (EPA), but the benefits – particularly late in the course of an illness – appear at best marginal. The endpoint of any intervention in this setting is improved survival, function and comfort. Without being able to predictably influence any of these, changes in laboratory parameters alone (such as total weight) mean little in real terms to most people with a life-limiting illness. The need to address the systemic insult that is threatening homeostasis remains the key to providing better global outcomes that are valued by the person and their family. It appears that at least in some end-stage settings, obesity may provide a protective factor against cachexia.[21]

## Medications

Several medications have been extensively studied in a bid to reverse cachexia. These include progestational agents, cannabinoids, glucocorticoids, thalidomide and eicosapentaenoic acid (EPA).

Progestational agents have been studied in randomized controlled trials against placebo, glucocorticoids and anabolic corticosteroids.[22] Although there may be gains in total weight, the benefits are marginal in terms of objective improvements in functional status or in survival.[14] Cannabinoids are used to improve appetite. In so doing, they are reflecting the social and cultural well-being associated with food. This again contrasts with changing function or survival. The side-effects of these medications, particularly dysphoria, limit their use overall. Glucocorticoids are frequently used in practice to try to reduce the day-to-day impact of cachexia. However, their use is associated with significant morbidity (e.g. proximal myopathy, glucose intolerance, frank diabetes, profound depression and hypomania). Weight gained is predominantly water and adipose tissue, and there are no data to support improvements in lean body mass.

More recently, interest has focused on the benefits of thalidomide and EPA to modulate weight loss. Thalidomide is being tested in randomized studies. EPA may well have a dose–response relationship to improving lean body mass in people with advanced cancer.[7] It is early days, and any benefit needs to be distinguished from anti-tumor effects, especially for the anti-angiogenic agent thalidomide, but arresting lean body mass seems achievable in the short term.[23,24]

## Attitudinal changes

There is great interest in the connection between body and mind at the end of life. Does a positive attitude have an impact on survival? Does trying to induce a positive attitude in someone who is negative improve function, comfort or survival? Positive attitude is a factor so many anxious relatives would like to believe makes a difference. There is conflicting evidence. There are population data to support the idea that time of death is influenced by factors other than the disease, but the data are currently not there to inform a reproducible answer. This is not to say there are no measures that can demonstrate differences in key neuroimmunological pathways with positive thinking, but whether this translates to the big-picture changes patients value is not clear.

## Local, comorbid and systemic effects

### Local effects from the primary cause of the life-limiting illnesses

In a minority of people with a life-limiting illness, a single organ system will fail and in turn lead to death. End-stage chronic organ failure with a predictable progression is more likely to manifest itself as a systemic problem than as local disease. The person with gradually worsening single-organ function may well die as a result of acute worsening of function due to a specific insult. For example, a person with severe emphysema could die from an acute bacterial chest infection. Even in this setting, the systemic responses that can adequately match the insult are likely to be already compromised. As such, it should be considered that systemic factors have failed to maintain homeostasis.

By contrast, someone with acute organ failure may well die as a result of this. Single-organ function may be compromised by direct local pathology, such as obstruction of major airways, the biliary tree, the gastrointestinal tract, the central nervous system (CNS) circulation of cerebrospinal fluid, or ureters by intra-luminal or extrinsic compression. Such obstruction directly impairs the functioning of the organ system affected, and causes secondary dysfunction from infection, pain, dyspnea, changing CNS function or vomiting, depending on the system affected. Death can occur rapidly without the usual warning signs of a progressive systemic decline in activities of daily living, weight, appetite and energy. Acute single-organ failure is also the setting in which it is most likely there will be the potential for an aspect of the acute pathology that can be reversed, especially if this person was otherwise systemically reasonably well.

### Comorbid illnesses at the end of life

The other issue that can confound the care of someone with an advanced, progressive life-limiting illness is the best way to manage long-term comorbidities. These comorbid illnesses can contribute to the progressive morbidity if not actively managed. Medication metabolism can change. Exaggerated effects of medications can occur as the result of higher serum levels because of changed metabolism, reduced excretion, or changed volume of distribution. Drugs with a narrow therapeutic window need careful monitoring in this setting.

Some comorbid illnesses will likely improve at the end of life; for example, hypertension or insulin resistance in type II diabetes mellitus may well be improved as a collateral effect of the systemic weight loss of disease progression. Other single-organ problems, such as azotemia, where continued adequate hydration is essential, may worsen with decreasing or erratic fluid intake late in the course of the disease.

Clarity about what is being treated or prevented is a key basis for the continued prescribing of medication for long-term comorbid conditions. Clearly, tertiary prevention is likely to need to continue later into a life-limiting illness than primary prevention. Likewise, if the benefits of treatment are measured over many years in hundreds of people to avoid one adverse event, then there is a strong case for ceasing that medication before it causes morbidity or adverse medication interactions.[25]

## Systemic and local effects that explain frequently encountered symptoms

### Fatigue

Fatigue is the most frequently encountered symptom in the disease progression of life-limiting illnesses. Although there may be reversible intercurrent causes (anemia, hypothyroidism), without a discrete reversible cause it is unlikely that fatigue can be directly treated. As outlined, fatigue is a cardinal systemic manifestation of the factors that mediate disease progression. Energy conservation is a cornerstone of minimising the impact of this symptom. Graded exercise may have a role in people with better functional status earlier in the disease trajectory.

### Pain

As a complex somato-sensory experience, pain is as much the insult as the interpretation and response. For many people, the underlying etiology of pain is clearly defined from history, examination and investigations. Like all pain, the ultimate interpretation of the symptom is a highly individual response to a complex set of circumstances. For many people, pain may seem out of proportion to the pathology that can be demonstrated. For some the perception is far greater than the insult demonstrated and for others apparently much less. This variation makes the person's history *the* key component in the evaluation of pain. Although potential mechanisms causing pain are important to consider (distension, distortion, ischemia, inflammation, infection, fracture, raised intra-cranial pressure, invasion and compression of nerves), so is the meaning of the pain to this person in the context of their life – past, present and future.

### Nausea

Nausea is a series of sensations commonly felt to reflect the possibility of vomiting. (There are a group of people for whom the key manifestation of problems is vomiting without warning – raised intracranial pressure or very proximal gastro-intestinal tract obstructions are common causes of vomiting without nausea.) Although the major causes are broadly grouped under CNS, upper gastrointesti-nal pathology (including hepatic pathology), metabolic (especially uremia), medications, and vestibular dysfunction, a clear relationship with symptomatic interventions is still theoretical.[26]

As with most symptoms in a progressive life-limiting illness, the etiology of nausea is usually multi-factorial. Even when a likely cause has been identified, in most people with progressive disease, polypharmacy and metabolic dysfunctions are likely to contribute independently to the symptom of nausea.

## Dyspnea

Dyspnea, like fatigue, tends to worsen as the life-limiting illness progresses. Like nausea, dyspnea is almost always multi-factorial. The inanition of cachexia weakens the muscles of respiration as it weakens all muscles in the body. The ability to respond adequately to infection is systemically challenged by less robust cellular and humoral immunity. Although progressively impaired gas exchange may occur in relation to the primary life-limiting illness, it can also be as a result of superimposed pulmonary thrombo-embolic disease, arrhythmias, or left-sided cardiac failure.

## Constipation

Constipation is frequently attributed to the use of opioids in people with a life-limiting illness. There are, however, other contributing factors – changes in oral intake and food preferences, less mobility and (often) compromised fluid intake. The multi-factorial etiology of a symptom means the clinician needs to reverse those components that are amenable to treatment, and rely on symptomatic treat-ment for the other factors. For most people these two processes need to occur simultaneously. It is also a process of diminishing returns – the most benefit is likely to be gained early in trying to ameliorate the symptom.

## Translating the science into frequently asked questions
### Questions from patients
*'How will I die?'*

Most people want, at some stage, to talk about the process of dying if they have a life-limiting illness. When asking the question, for many people it will be based on other people they have encountered (often through the period of diagnosis and treatment of people who have the same illness) and perceptions of the processes of dying they have witnessed more broadly. (There is also a group of people who have had little or nothing to do with death in their entire life). The question is especially poignant for people with lung cancer or pulmonary fibrosis, who fear they will suffocate; people with fungating head and neck cancers, who may have had a 'sentinel' bleed; or people with upper gastrointestinal cancers, who fear they will exsanguinate.

For most people with a life-limiting illness, such specific causes of death are unlikely. It is far more likely that death will be the progression of systemic whole-body close-down – the 'final common pathway'.

### 'How long have I got?'

For most people with a life-limiting illness, the disease progression is predictable. Factors that indicate systemic change include energy levels, weight and appetite. The rate of change in level of function gives a clear indication of the time people have left.

## Questions from caregivers

### 'Won't hydration or nutrition help?'

Weight loss and loss of energy are not due to poor nutritional intake, but result from inadequate nutritional uptake at a cellular level, mediated by, among other things, cytokines. Additional caloric or protein intake in established cachexia does not change the prognosis, the course of the disease, or the person's function or comfort.

### 'Why doesn't he/she exercise more? He/she needs to get up and around'

Further diminishing energy reserves in established cachexia by exercising has not been shown to make a positive change to the course of the illness. Catabolism is not reversed with exercise in progressive end-stage disease.

## References

1 Conraads VM, Bosmans JM, Vrints CJ. Chronic heart failure: an example of a systemic chronic inflammatory disease resulting in cachexia. *Int J Cardiol.* 2002; **85**: 33–49.
2 Hack V, Schmid D, Breitkreutz R, *et al.* Cystine levels, cystine flux, and protein catabolism in cancer cachexia, HIV/SIV infection, and senescence. *FASEB J*; **11**: 84–92.
3 Yeh S-S, Schuster MW. Geriatric cachexia: the role of cytokines. *Am J Clin Nutr.* 1999; **70**: 183–97.
4 Kotler DP. Cachexia. *Ann Intern Med.* 2000; **133**: 622–34.

5  Debigare R, Cote CH, Maltais F. Peripheral muscle wasting in chronic obstructive pulmonary disease. *Am J Respir Crit Care Med.* 2001; **164**: 1712–17.

6  Witte KK, Clark AL. Nutritional abnormalities contributing to cachexia in chronic disease. *Int J Cardiol.* 2002; **85**: 23–31.

7  Fearon KCH, von Meyenfeldt MF, Moses AGW, *et al.* Effect of a protein and energy dense n-3 fatty acid enriched oral supplement on loss of weight and lean tissue in cancer cachexia: a randomised double blind trial. *Gut.* 2003; **52**: 1479–86.

8  Fearon KCH, Borland W, Preston T, *et al.* Cancer cachexia: influence of systemic ketosis on substrate levels and nitrogen metabolism. *Am J Clin Nutr.* 1988; **47**: 42–8.

9  Cahlin C, Korner A, Axelsson H, *et al.* Experimental cancer cachexia: the role of host-derived cytokines interleukin (IL)-6, IL12, interferon-gamma, and tumour necrosis factor alpha evaluated in gene knockout, tumour bearing mice on C57 B1 background and eicosanoid-dependent cachexia. *Canc Res.* 2000; **60**: 5488–93.

10  Rubin H. Cancer cachexia: its correlations and causes. *Proc Natl Acad Sci.* 2003; **100**: 5384–9.

11  Grimble RF. Nutritional therapy for cancer cachexia. *Gut.* 2003; **52**: 1391–2.

12  Morrison SD. Origins of anorexia in neoplastic disease. *Am J Clin Nutr.* 1978; **31**: 1104–7.

13  Davis MP. Eicosapentaenoic acid: the answers are not all in. *J Clin Oncol.* 2005; **23**: 3854.

14  Jatoi A, Kumar S, Sloan JA, *et al.* On appetite and its loss. *J Clin Oncol.* 2000; **18**: 2930–2.

15  Brennan MF. Total parenteral nutrition in the cancer patient. *N Eng J Med.* 1981; **305**: 375–82.

16  Berry C, Clark AL. Catabolism in chronic heart failure. *Eur Heart J.* 2000; **21**: 521–32.

17  Sharma R, Anker SD. Cytokines, apoptosis and cachexia: the potential for TNF antagonism. *Int J Cardiol.* 2002; **85**: 161–71.

18  Anker SD, Volterrani M, Pflaum CD, *et al.* Acquired growth hormone resistance in patients with chronic heart failure: implications for therapy with growth hormone. *J Am Coll Cardiol.* 2001; **38**: 443–52.

19  Filippatos GS, Anker SD, Kremastinos DT. Pathophysiology of peripheral muscle wasting in cardiac cachexia. *Curr Op Clin Nutr Metabol Care.* 2005; **8**: 249–54.

20  Filippatos GS, Kanatselos C, Manolatos DD, *et al.* Studies on apoptosis and fibrosis in skeletal musculature: a comparison of heart failure patients with and without cardiac cachexia. *Int J Cardiol.* 2003; **90**: 107–13.

21  Davos CH, Doehner W, Rauchhaus M, *et al.* Body mass index and survival in patients with chronic heart failure without cachexia: the importance of obesity. *J Cardiac Fail.* 2003; **9**: 29–35.

22  Loprinzi CL, Kugler JW, Sloan JA, *et al.* Randomised comparison of megestrol acetate versus dexamethasone versus fluoxymesterone for the treatment of cancer anorexia/cachexia. *J Clin Oncol.* 1999; 3299–306.

23  Gordon JN, Green SR, Goggin PM. Cancer cachexia. *QJM.* 2005; **98**: 779–88.

24  Gordon JN, Trebble TM, Ellis RD, *et al.* Thalidomide in the treatment of cancer cachexia: a randomised placebo controlled trial. *Gut.* 2005; **54**: 540–5.

25  Stevenson J, Miller C, Abernethy AP, *et al.* Management of long-term comorbidities in the setting of end stage disease. *BMJ* 2004; **329**: 909–12.

26  Glare P, Kristjanson L. Systematic review of the efficacy of antiemetics in the treatment of nausea in patients with far-advanced cancer. *Support Care Canc.* 2004; **12**: 432–40.

## Selected texts describing symptom pathophysiology, control and management

Doyle G, Hanks G, MacDonald N, editors. *Oxford Textbook of Palliative Medicine*. Oxford, New York: Oxford University Press; 1998.

Regnard C, Hockley J. *A Guide to Symptom Relief in Palliative Care*. 5th ed. Oxford: Radcliffe Medical Press; 2004.

Woodruff, R. *Palliative Medicine: evidence-based symptomatic and supportive care for patients with advanced cancer*. 4th ed. Melbourne: Oxford University Press; 2004.

# CHAPTER 4

# Life-limiting illness: the illness experience

*DAVID SEAMARK, CLARE SEAMARK, JENNY HYNSON*

## Introduction

In the previous chapter the physiological events of dying were examined. Here the intertwined personal perceptions of the dying process are described.

The chapter has two sections – one deals with the adult experience, and the second describes that of the child who is dying. The first is written by Drs David and Clare Seamark, GPs who practice in rural England. They have spent many years researching the experience of people with life-limiting illness, in particular non-malignant illness.

While there are many aspects of these experiences common to both children and adults, the superimposed processes of emotional and psychological maturation in children create a completely different perspective to life-limiting conditions. Understanding this process will help practitioners to approach dying children appropriately. It will also help parents placed in this most difficult of circumstances to anticipate potential pitfalls in the way they approach their child. Dr Hynson is an Australian pediatrician who has specialized in the palliative care of children. (Her examination of the responses of parents and siblings to the dying child is found in the following chapter.)

## Section 1: The illness experience for adults

*David and Clare Seamark*

In writing this section we have used some of the literature relating to patients' experiences of palliative care. This has been complemented by our combined 35 years' experience working in a UK primary care setting and dealing on a day-to-day basis with people dying of both malignant and non-malignant illnesses. Although we have sourced studies from different parts of the world, much of our experience is obviously UK-based, as is that of the patients whose accounts we have included.

To give the real flavour of how it is for patients dying of both malignant and non-malignant disease, we also use two other sources. The first is from Harry, who was both a patient of our practice and a true and valued friend. The second voice is that of John Diamond, a professional London journalist, who developed what later turned out to be cancer of the tongue in 1997 and wrote both in his *Times* column and later a book about his experiences.

### Harry

Harry's widow Rosalind has given permission for Harry's story to be told, and indeed a full account with pictures can be found on Harry's website: http://www. hugo.uwclub.net/hmp/harry.htm.

Harry was born in pre-Second World War Austria, and his Jewish descent placed him and his family at high risk of persecution. The family fled Austria in 1939 to find sanctuary in Britain. An illustrious wartime career followed, during which he married Rosalind (after a courtship of days). A variety of careers including running a riding school led to Harry and Rosalind settling in rural Devon on the edge of a small medieval village. They had three children. One daughter farms nearby, the other daughter lives in Australia, and their son is in northern England. The social norm of cigarette smoking had consequences for Harry's health in later life.

Harry and (inevitably) Rosalind's illness experience was long and varied. The following pages will attempt to describe the various stages, through initial presentation, diagnosis, treatment and palliative care, drawing on Harry's personal account, his medical record and a transcript of an interview conducted towards the end of his life.

As is the case for an increasing number of patients, Harry was confronted with two life-threatening diagnoses: chronic obstructive pulmonary disease (COPD) and carcinoma of the rectum. The medical record first mentions COPD in 1976, and this was the condition that led to his death in May 2002 with a death certificate entry of 'exacerbation of COPD'. The rectal carcinoma was diagnosed in 1998, and this brought another set of challenges for Harry and Rosalind, their family and healthcare providers. We plan to compare and contrast the effects of living with a cancer diagnosis and life-threatening non-cancer diagnosis in this account. There are areas common to both, as well as differences that require recognition and a different approach by healthcare providers.

### John Diamond

John was a London journalist writing a regular column for the *Times* newspaper and contributing to radio and television programs in the 1990s. He had his first symptoms of the cancer in 1996 when in his mid-forties, and he wrote of this in his weekly *Times* column. Later he put his experiences into a book *Because Cowards Get Cancer Too . . .* He vividly and movingly describes some of the stages and experiences he went through as he and his family came to terms with the diagnosis and later terminal prognosis of his cancer.

At the time of his diagnosis he was married to Nigella with two very young children. John had been a heavy smoker in his younger days, but had substituted cigarette smoking for nicotine chewing gum in the 10 years before his cancer diagnosis. Extracts from his book are printed with the kind permission of the publishers.

## Receiving bad news

By definition, the receiving of bad news is a disturbing experience, and the literature on cancer and palliative care is full of accounts of bad news being poorly communicated (*see* http://www. Dipex.org.uk). This is partly the health professionals' fault, but account needs to be taken of the ability of patients and relatives to take in bad news at a time of heightened stress and anxiety. It is also important to remember that the patient already has an inkling that bad news is going to be broken – after all, they went to see the doctor in the first place because they thought there was something wrong. Harry describes how he was convinced that something *was* wrong, and how eventually this was confirmed.

> I had, of course, increasing health problems, and whenever something new happened, one was inclined to take it in one's stride. So I went to see the doctor a few months earlier to consult him about recurring shows of blood. He dismissed this with the explanation that I had piles. When eventually I produced a fairly substantial amount of blood, I said to myself that I would have to see the doctor again if this persisted. I am afraid it did and one day I had a considerable haemorrhage. This time the doctor took notice and referred me to the Royal Devon and Exeter Hospital. They took all sorts of tests and two days before our proposed party I was told I would have to go to hospital at once for an operation for cancer of the bowel. (*Harry's website*)

John Diamond had also been unwell for some time before his cancer was diagnosed. He clearly speaks from his own experience of having bad news broken to him and how whatever is said one always hears the worst.

> Mine was just a small local cancer, they said, and one that could be scared off with a little radiotherapy. It wasn't as it turned out, but it didn't matter for nobody receives a diagnosis of even the least invasive cancer with anything but fear and dread. ( *John Diamond*, p. 7)

> Tell anyone that you have cancer and what they'll hear is that you're about to die. Why would they not? It's what you heard when you got the diagnosis, after all. ( *John Diamond*, p. 8)

In healthcare systems organized around segregated family practice and specialist care, the giving of a cancer diagnosis is usually performed by the specialist, with the family practitioner often involved in the role of reiterating the diagnosis and explaining the plans for treatment.

The interaction between the family doctor and the patient is crucial and can produce an increased level of trust and openness that is beneficial later on in the illness journey. Considerable effort has been made in recent years to improve the breaking of bad news, building on the principle of of a number of multiple steps (e.g. ten or six), described by Kaye and others.[1,2]

These approaches aim to take the person breaking the bad news and the person/people receiving it through several stages. First, it is vital to have all the facts to hand and the right place to give the news. Then it is important to review what is already known or suspected. The doctor should determine how much information is wanted while allowing the patient to deal with it in their own way. It is necessary to find out what the patient's concerns are and to allow them to express their feelings. At the end of the consultation, an opportunity should be offered for further discussion in the patient's own time. It is important to engender some hope into the situation wherever possible.

The advantage a primary care physician may have is previous knowledge of the patient and their family. This prior knowledge can help in the pacing of the consultation and knowing when to tread lightly. Another advantage for the primary care physician is the ability to see the patient at more frequent intervals than the hospital-based clinician can. Consequently, the 10 steps may not be completed in one appointment, but can be reasonably extended over some days. John Diamond identified very clearly that there were steps in the information that he was given about both his illness and the treatment options, and calls this 'gradual disclosure'.

> For it was with radiotherapy that I would first discover the principle of gradual disclosure which almost all doctors practise.

The principle is simple and at first glance makes a certain sort of sense. In the case of complicated, possibly fatal and emotionally charged illness, never tell the patient more than he is likely to find out for himself, and only ever give the best-case scenario. Thus when we first talked about radiotherapy we were talking about a simple procedure with very few side-effects. When we were discussing occult sites for my primary tumour we were considering a place which almost certainly would not exist after radiotherapy. When some months along the line, the subject of surgery came up it was an in-and-out snip-snip sort of surgery.

But the radiotherapy turned out to have a mass of side-effects, it didn't kill the primary and it would lead to eight hours of major surgery. (*John Diamond*, pp. 63–4)

However, he is also asking for both the institutions and the professionals to do this and, as in Kaye's 10 steps, to engender hope:

The Marsden really is how hospitals should be run: intelligently, flexibly, always engendering hope. (*John Diamond*, p. 11)

Although consultation length in UK primary care in particular is frequently criticized, the cumulative effect of repeated consultations has been seen as advantageous and vital to a productive patient–doctor relationship.[3] The amount of contact Harry had with his GP is shown below. The contacts with his GP peaked during the time of initial diagnosis of his cancer and treatment for that, and progressively more telephone contacts were made with his GP as his condition deteriorated. There were also many largely unrecorded contacts with the district nurse and hospice domiciliary nurse on a weekly basis during the last two years of his life.

**TABLE 4.1** Recorded contacts with Harry over the last 10 years of his life

| YEAR | CONTACTS | YEAR | CONTACTS |
|------|----------|------|----------|
| 1992 | 9 | 1998 | 47 |
| 1993 | 10 | 1999 | 30 |
| 1994 | 12 | 2000 | 26 |
| 1995 | 18 | 2001 | 21 |
| 1996 | 24 | Up to May 2002 | 15 |
| 1997 | 49 | | |

When dealing with a non-malignant life-threatening illness, the issue of breaking bad news becomes somewhat clouded. The issue hinges on the question of prognosis and knowledge of disease progression. In Harry's case, mention of chronic respiratory disease was made many years before his death from the condition.

> My life then returned more or less to normal though emphysema continued to be a problem and the doctor told me it would never get better, but gradually get worse. I am afraid he was right and at the time of writing this, I am seriously handicapped. (*Harry's website, looking back to 1979*)

Interestingly, Harry took on board the concepts that his emphysema was chronic and progressive. These concepts extend to other non-malignant life-threatening disease such as heart failure and renal failure. The difficulties in communication for these illnesses center on problems of prognosis and the balance between active medical treatments and palliative treatments.

Literature derived from hospital-based studies often quotes prognosis in severe heart failure (New York Heart Association levels III–IV) being as limited as that of lung cancer. This is true. However, studies in primary care reveal a less aggressive disease course, which with modern management may extend life by years and may result in death from other causes.[4,5] So the primary care clinician is left in the position of deciding how much to discuss disease progression, possible symptoms and ultimate prognosis with a patient with chronic heart and lung disease.

There are clues from the literature about what patients' needs are. Remarkable similarities have been found among the perspectives of patients with COPD, AIDS and cancer, including the importance of emotional support, communication and accessibility, and continuity.[6] One study based in Scotland looked at patients with cancer. The vast majority (96%) wanted more information about their disease, and to know that it was cancer, their chance of cure and the side-effects of treatment.[7] Patients with COPD wanted patient education in five areas: diagnosis and disease process, treatment, prognosis, what dying might be like, and advance care planning. For patients with AIDS, pain control was a dominant theme, and for patients with cancer maintaining hope despite a terminal prognosis was prominent.

Advance care planning (which can include the preparation of living wills/ advance directives, together with treatment options) has been implemented in the USA, with some positive outcomes in terms of patient satisfaction, increased incidence of deaths at home and use of hospice services.[8,9] How such initiatives might transfer to other healthcare settings is uncertain.[10] Qualitative interviews with patients with end-stage COPD and their carers in the UK revealed a desire for better information sharing and surveillance of care.[11] This surveillance role might be carried out by the primary healthcare team, or with the help of specialist respiratory and hospice services.

John Diamond expressed his appreciation that he was being followed up and that people were looking out for any new problems for him.

> But as long as I was seeing one Marsden person I had access to them all. Any dropped

> hint of remission, of pain, of something slightly dodgy would get me an instant referral
> to the sanctuary of a Rhys Evans or a Breach or a Henk. ( *John Diamond*, p. 226)

The receiving of bad news does not end with what the patient is told; the patient may then have to go and tell relatives and friends. This can be particularly difficult when telling parents, because they often feel very upset and that it seems the wrong way round for the child to be ill or die first. In past generations doctors often used to tell the relatives first and the news was kept from the patient in the mistaken belief that it was better for them not to know. If they did know it might hasten their death. Fallowfield and colleagues have shown that although this was often done with good intentions, communication is very important in palliative care. The truth about their condition is likely to upset someone, but being kept in the dark is worse.[12] Research such as this has brought considerable changes, certainly in British medicine, with the patient almost always being the first to be informed and the relatives only told with the patient's consent. At times, though, the patient may prefer health professionals to break the news to their relatives rather than do it themselves.

### Patients' decisions and involvement in treatment and curative options

Many people when they are given the diagnosis of cancer immediately see their own death. The health professional imparting the news may then offer the prospect of cure from surgery or medical treatment. The extent to which patients wish to be involved in their own treatment and decision-making choices can vary. It would appear that people desire more information about their condition than doctors think they want, but this does not necessarily translate into a desire to participate in the decision-making process regarding treatment.[13] The information given may be inadequate and lack an accurate, objective appraisal of what the treatment will actually be like. Most patients want to know their diagnosis and treatment options and side-effects, and usually they want these to be communicated by a hospital doctor.[7]

Here, useful websites such as CancerBACUP, Dipex and NeLH may add a subjective dimension to an evidence-based medical model of treatment. It is also possible that decisions will change with the illness.[13] People may be more likely to accept heroic attempts at cure early on, but less likely to accept treatments that will affect their quality of life when cure is no longer possible.[14]

> . . . but this time we all seemed to understand that the odds had changed.
>
> Changing odds must be the unchanging condition at the Marsden. For so long now one of the thoughts which had sustained me was that however terrible a state some of the people I saw at the hospital looked to be in, somebody here, somebody who knew about cancer reckoned it worth their while trying to find the right treatment.

> . . . I understood how often the staff here must see somebody turn up for their first
> treatment unscarred, full of life and substance, and return again and again, each time
> less vital, less hopeful, each time the odds slightly lower. ( *John Diamond*, p. 198)

In women with breast cancer, the importance of effective communication about
the diagnosis and treatment options helps with the long-term adjustment to the
treatment. The desire for autonomy among these women may be less strong than
the need for clear and accurate information. In a study looking at how women
responded to different surgeons' approaches and the chance to share in decision-
making, only 20% of women wanted an active role and half the women wanted
the surgeon to make the decision. It is important that as well as being given
enough information, patients are also given the right to decline the opportunity
to participate in decision-making.[15] Some people will have very strong ideas about
treatments they may or may not agree to have, though again these can change
with the course of the illness. Early on John Diamond had been determined that
he should not lose his tongue in the heroic surgery proposed. Later he thought
this might have been a futile gesture.

Harry's story brings us to consider the experience of not only receiving bad
news, but also having to cope with the prospect of disfiguring surgery, living with
an ostomy and having radiotherapy. For many patients, the diagnosis of cancer is
accompanied by a plethora of information, appointments and treatments that can
cause disruption and bewilderment to the patient and the whole family. Efforts
have been made in recent years to integrate the delivery of such complex care with
specialist nurses and patient advocates. Harry's experience was positive in that the
consultant fitted in with plans to celebrate his Golden Wedding anniversary.

> They took all sorts of tests and two days before our proposed party I was told I would
> have to go to hospital at once for an operation for cancer of the bowel. The surgeon
> was an extremely understanding and helpful man, and I asked him could this not wait
> a few days until after our party, and he agreed without hesitation. I did not let it spoil
> things, and gave it very little thought until it actually happened. (*Harry's website*)

In many ways the initial treatments for malignant diseases can seem worse than
the cancer as it presents. In this way malignant disease may differ from the non-
cancer terminal illness. Although patients with COPD and heart failure may
have had a lot of medical treatments, they are less likely to have experienced
mutilating surgery for their condition, or to have undergone radiotherapy or
chemotherapy.

Both the patients and their clinicians may underestimate the effects of the
treatment involved. However, the practice of 'gradual disclosure' that John
Diamond has described comes into play here, probably because knowing the
very worst at the start might make going through with any treatment even more

unbearable. The treatments can be both distressing and leave the patient with a mutilated or different body.

Here Harry describes his experience.

> A few days after we celebrated our Golden Wedding, I entered hospital and had quite a big operation called colostomy. It took some getting used to the idea of having one's body mutilated. Strangely enough my memory is a little hazy from that point onwards. I had some time in Exeter and was then sent back to Honiton Hospital [community hospital] for post-operative care. I cannot remember how long for. When finally I was discharged I had to be taken to Exeter daily for six weeks for radiotherapy. Quite a task for Rosalind, but we accepted it as inevitable. The purpose of the treatment was to shrink the tumour sufficiently to make it ready for a really thorough operation to remove all the bits and pieces, which had been affected by cancer. I believe I am right in saying that operation took place in October that year and was rather bigger than the first one. (*Harry's website*)

John Diamond also describes the effect of his treatments on his physical form.

> The problem with major surgery – any surgery – is that there is no real way of anyone telling you how it will be when you come round. I'd had conversations with various of the medical people and although nobody goes into any great details about the tubes and the bed, I had some idea of the wreckage that my physical form would suffer – that I'd be cut, and bandaged, and scarred. And, I'd guessed that I'd feel pretty miserable, although misery wasn't really the term to describe the mixture of drug-dampened pain, irritation and physical constraint. But nobody can tell you how it feels to be that post-operative person, the person who is lying there waiting for the new chapter to start and with no idea of how that chapter will read. I knew that everything that had been done to me would have a permanent effect, but I couldn't say what effect – on my constitution, my looks, my voice, my career, my persona – would be. I lay there and contemplated the new me and was frustrated by the shallowness of contemplation that was possible. (*John Diamond*, pp. 158–9)

As we have seen, the effects of cancer treatment will often seem worse than the experience of the disease so far. The decisions made about the treatment will also be affected by the stage of the illness. When John Diamond found that his cancer was still there he was expecting to have a bigger operation, but found that it was too late for that.

> If I leave the cancer to take its natural course I have about six months left. If I have chemotherapy, and assuming the chemotherapy works in my case and that it's not so arduous as to be unbearable, then I might double or treble that time and there's a small but significant chance of my doing even better than that given that the cancers are tiny and I feel healthier than I ever have. I'll take the chemotherapy, of course. Why would I not? (*John Diamond*, p. 254)

## Losses and adaptations in palliative care

The sense of loss is something that comes across from patients with a terminal condition. This loss has many aspects. Ultimately it will be the loss of their life, but in the time before that it can mean many other losses, such as employment and financial, health and a whole body, social life, relationships, and of the life not lived. This sense of loss is to some extent tempered by the adaptations people make.

Both Harry and John Diamond have described how they felt their bodies were changed and mutilated by the treatments they endured. These effects may be different in patients with a purely non-malignant condition, but increasing breathlessness and frailty can lead to a feeling that your body is no longer one you know or can rely on. This idea that you are now a different person came through in both Harry's and John Diamond's accounts.

> When I finally got back home we had to accept the fact that I was now fairly seriously disabled. (*Harry's website*)

> We drove home and lay together in our bed for what was to be the last time as the couple we have been for eight years. Tomorrow I would become somebody else. (*John Diamond*, p. 144)

For patients with COPD, losses related to undertaking even the most basic of daily activities were felt most keenly. (The following quotations come from the authors' qualitative data set of patients with terminal COPD. Names have been changed to protect anonymity, apart from Harry's.)

> I even have a job to undress myself, or dress myself. I have to struggle to undress and dress for everything. (*Cliff*)

Harry also described this loss from his COPD.

> A complete loss of personal liberty and now I can't walk, I can't do anything. (*Harry*)

However, he then goes on to describe his attitude to adapting to this situation.

> I think far more along the lines of 'can do' rather than along the lines of what is impossible to do. (*Harry*)

Others described these losses, and, particularly if they were younger, how it also affected their employment.

> It stopped everything in its tracks [had to stop work], yeah change of lifestyle completely from a doer to a non-doer. And the simplest tasks now are a big effort. (*Gordon*)

Losses relating to social life were very common in patients with COPD as they found it to difficult to go out. Sometimes they didn't even have enough breath to talk to other people. Harry explained how some of his relationships became 'telephone friendships' as he used that as an alternative to going out himself.

One of the other themes was of losses of a life that had previously been expected. Obviously this affected partners and other members of the family as well.

> We had a lot of ideas, but you know, ill health messed it all up. That's life for you. (*Gordon*)

> When we were first married we couldn't afford to do the things we wanted to do, now we can and I've got this damn thing. (*Henry*)

> I find it hard with my granddaughter. I can't go out in the garden and kick a ball around with her and throw her around and play . . . like most grandfathers do. (*Gordon*)

Adaptive difficulties related to financial problems, and being unable to change to a sedentary life and the accompanying boredom. This also affected their carers, who were often deeply enmeshed with the illness as well.

## Transition to non-curative and palliative care

Primary care teams have long experience of providing non-curative, palliative and end-of-life care to patients in the community. The concept of a gradual transition between curative care and non-curative palliative care has been taken on board in the UK setting by both specialist and generalist palliative care health professionals. These two groups share values of holistic, and patient- and family-centered care based where possible in the community. Problems can still arise when the disease trajectory is prolonged and the prognosis uncertain, as is often the case with a non-malignant diagnosis such as terminal organ failure illness. The differing trajectories of cancer and non-cancer illnesses are illustrated in Figure 4.1.

The need to move from 'prognostic paralysis' to active total care, especially for patients with chronic illness, has recently been discussed.[15] Ways of tackling the problem of ascertaining who is in need of palliative care are being actively researched. The development of cancer and chronic disease registers in primary care is a start, especially if prognosis can be refined by simple clinical scoring scales. A clinician asking the question, 'Would I be surprised if my patient were to die in the next 12 months?' is perhaps more useful than stating a definite prognosis, and could reasonably be employed by primary health care professionals.[16] With cancer, the realization that the cancer is no longer likely to be 'curable' may come at a more specific point in time, and John Diamond graphically describes this point of transition.

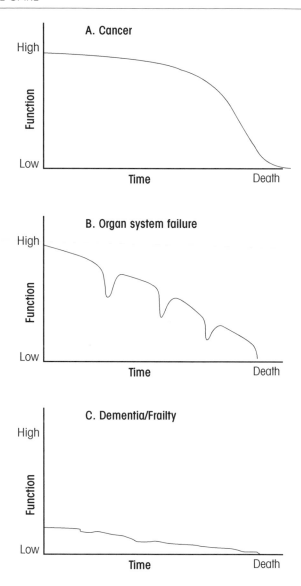

**FIGURE 4.1** The differing trajectories of cancer and non-malignant illnesses

Source: Lynn J, 2001[16]

But as soon as we arrived at the outpatients clinic we knew it was all up. Normally, and despite BUPA's* hefty chequebook, we conduct our clinical meetings in an ordinary white cubicle in the general outpatient's clinic; this time the receptionist gave us a tight smile and said Mr Rhys Evans had asked for us to be shown over to one of the chain-hotel designed consulting rooms in the Marsden's private wing. You do not ask for your patients to be taken to the comfy chairs if you're about to tell them that after all the shadow on the scan was a packet of Woodbines left on the machine by one of the cleaners.

When Rhys Evans arrived it was with the unspoken hint of worse news still. The list of clinical possibilities thus far have all been either surgical or radiological and I've known for some time that if a medical doctor ever turned up to a consultation then we were no longer talking about cure but about remission. Accompanying my surgeon were two men I'd not met before: a consultant medical oncologist and his registrar. Standing behind them, looking embarrassed, was a tallish man in hood and gown with a scythe over his shoulder.

Statistics tell us that anyone whose job is treating those diagnosed as having cancer will, in around 60% of cases, eventually have to dole out the worst possible news, and you'd suppose that after some years of doing it most doctors would find a way somewhere between the mawkish and the unnecessarily brusque which would serve them comfortably in the majority of cases. I suppose it's testimony to Peter Rhys Evans that he gave us the news white-faced, nervous, with eyes downcast. Much as he must have given the news the first time he ever had to, as if it were something both unsayable and already said. (*John Diamond*, pp. 253–4) (* a private health insurance fund)

In non-malignant conditions the time of transition can be more difficult to identify. GP discussion of prognosis with patients with severe COPD has been explored through survey and interview techniques. A survey of London GPs indicated that although a majority acknowledged a need to discuss prognosis, this was not actually reflected in their reported behaviour, with only 41% often or always discussing prognosis. It appeared that uncertainty among GPs as to how patients view the discussion of prognosis and inadequate preparation were potential barriers.[10]

Interviews with GPs in New Zealand produced a number of strategies that were used, or could be used, to facilitate discussion of prognosis with patients with COPD. These include awareness of the implications of diagnosis, use of uncertainty to ease discussion, beginning discussion early in the disease course, and identifying and using opportunities to discuss prognosis, such as after an exacerbation of the disease or a hospital admission.[17]

Are the palliative care needs of patients with a malignant diagnosis versus a non-malignant diagnosis really that different? In Harry's case, both life-threatening conditions co-existed and this is the situation for increasing numbers of patients as the population ages. His respiratory condition was progressing, but he also had the cancer and effects of treatment for that to contend with.

When I finally got back home we had to accept the fact that I was now fairly seriously disabled. Strangely enough the cancer gave me less trouble than my chest, which had deteriorated as a result of anaesthetics used for the two operations. For many weeks the District Nurse had to call daily to deal with the dressings. Social Services were wonderful and supplied all manner of appliances. Particularly helpful was an air mattress, which was like a cow's udder with thousands of teats, inflated by an electric motor. Pressure was electronically monitored, and if the thing went wrong an alarm blew your head off, and something had to be done about it. I don't remember what had to be done, but of course I was condemned to lying on my wound which was a bit sore, hence that mattress. (*Harry's website*)

Patients with life-threatening illness do experience spiritual and existential distress long before they die,[18] and being 'known' by your GP or community nurse is frequently found to be an important source of support in end-of-life care.[19] Evidence from real life indicates that patients who died with cardio-respiratory disease were less likely to be in receipt of formally identified terminal care and were likely to have had fewer drugs prescribed for palliation than patients with malignant disease; yet those with cardio-respiratory disease made similar demands on primary care teams and are likely to have unmet needs with respect to symptom palliation.[20] A comparison between patients with end-stage COPD and lung cancer in the UK found that patients with COPD had significantly impaired quality of life and emotional well-being, which may not be as well catered for in patients with lung cancer, nor do they receive holistic care appropriate to their needs.[21]

A study of GPs and specialists in the UK to determine their views about palliative care for heart failure yielded a sobering picture of poor-quality care for patients and frustration among doctors.[22] This study identified that predicting the illness trajectory is much harder in severe heart failure than in cancer and creates uncertainty in doctors, impeding the planning of appropriate care and of discussing prognosis. A community-based study from Scotland comparing illness trajectories, needs and service use of patients with lung cancer and patients with severe heart failure confirmed that care for people with advanced progressive illness is currently prioritized by diagnosis rather than need.[23] Patients with heart failure had a different illness trajectory from the more linear and predictable course of patients with lung cancer. Patients with heart failure had less information about and poorer understanding of their condition and prognosis, and were less involved in decision-making. Frustration, progressive losses, social isolation and the stress of balancing and maintaining a complex medication regimen dominated the lives of patients with heart failure. For patients with lung cancer and their carers, the prime concern was facing death. Heart failure patients received fewer health, social and palliative care services than patients with lung cancer, though in both groups care was often poorly co-ordinated.

An American perspective of palliative care for patients with heart failure has recently been published.[24] This draws attention to the need to consider – and if possible discuss – prognosis and advance directives. The issue of hospice care in the USA differs somewhat from that in the rest of the world because there is a requirement for a prognosis of less than six months to qualify for a hospice program. However, such a requirement may promote discussions around end-of-life care.

## Patients' experiences of difficult symptoms

Other chapters of this book deal with the pathophysiology and palliation of symptoms. Here we explore the subjective experience of symptoms. A number of studies have examined reported symptoms for patients dying from COPD.[11,25,26] Breathlessness, anxiety and panic are consistently reported as being intrusive and difficult to control. These symptoms are also common to those suffering from terminal heart failure and respiratory cancers.

Harry explains symptoms of breathlessness.

> Well I've been short of breath since I was about 40, but it has never been given a label of emphysema until about 15–20 years ago and then it was, it was put to me that it won't get better, it will get gradually worse, which it has. (*Harry's interview*)

> A complete loss of personal liberty and now I can't walk, I can't do anything, I think it's very claustrophobic, if I get these coughing bouts which I do get and really get terribly out of breath as a result then it's very frightening, very very frightening, and very inhibiting. (*Harry's interview*)

Other patients graphically describe their dyspnea and associated fear and anorexia linked to breathlessness. (Quotations come from the authors' qualitative data set of patients with COPD with the identities changed.)

> Can you imagine someone having a bag over their head? They're fighting for their breath. That's me, that is me, that is. (*Irvin*)

> I did say to him, 'You know this man that has run the London marathon in a deep sea diver's suit'. I said, 'I'm like that.' It takes all my strength pushing myself into a walk. (*Ernest*)

> No, one downfall of this thing, is you go off your food for a start, and you don't fancy nothing and you find you can't swallow so much as you'd like to swallow, you know, your throat get choked. (*Donald*)

In the UK, the Regional Study of Care for the Dying has investigated symptoms in terminal heart disease.[27] People who died from heart disease, including heart failure, had experienced a wide range of symptoms, often distressing and often lasting for more than six months. In addition to dyspnea, pain, nausea, constipation and low mood were common and poorly controlled. At least one in five had symptoms as severe as those in patients with cancer managed by specialist palliative care services. Pain affected 78% of patients in the UK study,[28] and in the USA the SUPPORT study reported severe symptoms in patients with heart failure, with 65% being breathless and 42% having severe pain.[29] The need to apply the lessons learnt from cancer palliative care to those patients dying of heart failure has also been highlighted.[30]

## The last days

Care of the dying patient has recently been the subject of a helpful review.[31] This emphasizes the challenge of transferring best practice from a hospice setting to other care settings, the importance of diagnosing dying, and the need for resources to enable patients to die with dignity in the place of their choice. A major initiative in the UK has been the promotion of the Macmillan Gold Standards Framework throughout primary care organizations.[32] The framework aims to support and facilitate the primary health care team towards highest-quality care for patients with any illness in the last stages of life.

Primary healthcare teams provide much of the medical care required by patients who die in the community. Although only about a quarter of patients die at home,[33] 90% of the care is delivered at home by GPs and primary care teams.[34] Although great progress in the development of palliative medicine as a speciality has been made throughout the world, the likelihood of all care of dying patients being taken over by specialists is remote. As a result, primary care teams will continue to be key providers of palliative care, particularly for the increasing population of elderly patients suffering from non-malignant terminal illness.[35]

How well do GPs deliver palliative care? This has been the subject of a systematic review,[19] salient points of which are discussed here. GPs' exposure to palliative care is small but consistent, with around five to fifteen cases per year being cared for, and there is evidence that GPs value this part of their work. Nurses have the most contact with palliative care patients at home, and when GPs and primary care work well the medical system as a whole works more efficiently, with some improvements in outcomes.

In spite of evidence of enhanced patient outcomes from GP participation in palliative care teams, the performance of GPs in delivering optimal pain and symptom control is questioned: reported pain and symptom control by GPs is somewhat worse than for practitioners caring for patients in inpatient units. This finding needs to be weighed against evidence of improvements over time in GP knowledge and practice of pain and symptom control, while acknowledging problems still exist with psychological aspects.

The need for team working was illustrated by a UK study that investigated barriers to adequate symptom control in palliative care by surveying the views of patients, GPs and community nurses on symptom control.[36] GPs and community nurses differed greatly in the symptoms they felt confident in controlling, and there was generally low agreement between patients' and GPs' reports of patient symptoms. GPs were most likely to miss symptoms that were perceived to be difficult to control, such as loss of appetitive, depression and bowel and bladder control, and that were less prevalent in the patient sample.

While acknowledging that the vast majority of care for the dying during their last year is provided at home, why is it that only 20 to 30% of patients of cancer actually die in their own home?[37] Although it is tempting to blame poor organization and lack of resources, the situation is not necessarily that simple. John Hinton's seminal work[34,38] involved closely examining the last months of life of a cohort of patients with cancer. Few patients living alone or with unfit relatives stayed at home, and the proportion of patients admitted to a hospice increased steadily with the duration of the illness. At this stage the patients' and carers' preferences also changed, with inpatient care becoming more favored. Initial assessment revealed a 100% preference for home care by patients and carers, but this fell steadily to 54% of patients and 45% of relatives as death approached. Reasons for the final admission were symptom control, the patient's deteriorated state and relatives needing relief. These final admissions were usually of short duration (30% were only one to three days) compared with the overall length of palliative care. At follow-up, relatives approved of where the patients had received care and died and often considered death as separate from the dying process and preferred it to happen in a hospice or hospital.

Clearly the preferences of patients and carers as to the place of death can change during the course of a terminal illness, and it is important for health professionals to elicit these preferences from time to time. The choices of where to die have also changed over recent years with the expansion of the hospice movement and the recognition of GP-led inpatients beds, such as in a UK community hospital, as alternatives to specialist hospice beds.[39,40]

In the UK currently, place of death for patients with cancer compared with place of death for all causes is as follows (*see* Table 4.2).

## What constitutes a good death?

Despite a recent increase in the attention given to improving end-of-life care, surprisingly little is understood about what constitutes a good death. A US survey of patients with cancer or HIV/AIDS, their families and health providers[42] identified six major components of a good death: pain and symptom management, clear decision-making, preparation for death, completion, contributing to others, and affirmation of the whole person. For each theme, biomedical psychological and spiritual components were identified, but physicians noticeably offered the most biomedical perspective. For patients and families, psychosocial and spiritual issues were as important as biomedical concerns.

**TABLE 4.2** Place of death in the UK

| PLACE OF DEATH | ALL DEATHS (%) | MALIGNANT NEOPLASM (%) |
|---|---|---|
| Hospital | 69.7 | 57.2 |
| Hospice | 4.4 | 15.7 |
| Other communal establishments; e.g. | | |
| nursing home | 7.6 | 3.3 |
| own home | 18.9 | 22.2 |
| other private house | 2.3 | 1.4 |

Source: www.statistics.gov.uk[41]

## How were these various themes played out in Harry's final illness?

The biomedical aspects of pain and symptom management were quite complex, along with the management of his comorbidities. Together with the COPD and colonic cancer, Harry also suffered from deafness, glaucoma, osteo-arthritis, prostatic hypertrophy, hiatus hernia symptoms, multiple pulmonary emboli requiring anti-coagulation, heart failure and recurrent depression. His list of prescribed medication was daunting, and the chances of drug interactions – particularly with his deteriorating physical condition – were high. The managing of comorbidities in patients at the end of life has recently been discussed,[43] emphasising the need to give due attention to both the patients' perceptions and the clinicians' responsibilities. Harry's GP and nursing team needed to make regular reviews of his symptom control and medication, and his clinical notes document frequent discussions with and correspondence from Harry on these issues.

The following are from letters from Harry to his GP.

> Depression seems to have been overcome, the bad sleeping only partly. On balance so far as I can see, things are not too bad.
>
> I remember how helpful the exercises were which I did in hospital. Would you be able to refer me to physio? Increased the oxygen from two litres to three. My gums are sore most of the time.

This is from a letter from Harry to the continence nurse.

> Daily blockages [of catheter] and very frequent bypasses. At times forgot to close the Flip-Flow valve after draining it and I wonder whether this could be another cause for the blockage. My wife doing a washout five times a week.

John Hinton found that 64% of patients he interviewed thought death certain and probable and 27% thought it possible. Interviewing Harry brought this response:

| | |
|---|---|
| *Interviewer:* | So how do you see the future? |
| *Harry:* | How do I see the future? – in a wooden box. |
| *Interviewer:* | So – it's a difficult question for me to ask you, but do you see this as a terminal illness? |
| *Harry:* | Yes. |
| *Interviewer:* | You don't see that there could be any cure? |
| *Harry:* | No, I've been told there aren't any. I'm not saying I shall die, but it's not an illness from which I hope to get better or be cured. |

The fact that the majority of patients realize they are dying can help prevent the community team entering a collusion of silence and denial that carers sometimes request in order to 'protect' the patient. This is not to say all patients wish to discuss their death, as illustrated by these accounts:

| | |
|---|---|
| *Interviewer:* | How do you view the future? |
| *Patient:* | I dread to think to be honest with you, I dread to think. I worry more about what is left behind. |
| *Interviewer:* | How do you view the future? |
| *Patient:* | Just want to live as long as I can. |
| *Interviewer:* | Do you think the illness will deteriorate? |
| *Patient:* | Well I've been told I'm never going to get better which hurts, but there you are, gotta swallow that one. |

For Harry and his wife Rosalind the illness experience had led to heightened spiritual awareness, which was seen as one positive outcome of the illness.

[The illness] has certainly made my spiritual awareness rather deeper than it used to be and spiritual output, or input if you like, has been very much increased by that; but I know I can't rely on myself nor anyone else to help me, but God. (*Harry*)

Harry's care was conducted at home for the majority of his final year of life, and it was his wish to die at home if possible. However, he required admissions to the local community hospital under the care of his GP to deal with exacerbations of his COPD and to provide respite for his wife. The role of UK community hospitals in palliative care has been explored, and there is evidence that medical care is comparable to that of inpatient hospices and that such hospitals can act as alternatives to hospice in more remote rural areas.[39,40]

In one study the availability of community hospital beds was associated with fewer deaths from cancer in a general hospital and allowed a greater proportion of patients to remain under the care of their GP.[44] The advantages of community hospital care include being cared for by staff known to the patient and carer, and ease of access. Disadvantages, when compared with hospice inpatient care, were problems of communication, shortage of nursing staff and lack of support in bereavement.[40]

Harry's final admission to the local community hospital came after a long night of discussion with Rosalind and the realization by both that she could not manage his care at home any longer. His last two weeks of life were spent under the care of his GP, with visits from the domiciliary specialist hospice nurse. He died peacefully with Rosalind and members of his family present.

How people deal with their impending death will vary as well. John Diamond describes quite clearly that although he knew he was dying, he wanted to live what life he had to the full and also think about his family's needs after he was gone.

> And so this is how you find me. Not quite waiting to die, because although I've accepted that I will, and sooner rather than later, the same rules apply to the foreshortened life as to the one of normal length: just as no well-balanced 45 year old says 'Why bother going to the movies? I'll be dead in 30 years' so I find that my imminent death doesn't stop me wanting to know what happens at the end of bad detective thrillers or wanting to spend time with Nigella and the children. Those things are still worth doing.
>
> As I write this we have all returned from buying a basket for the spaniel we are due to collect in a couple of days time. A friend e-mailed me when she heard this to tell me about how it's a denial of what's happening and what's about to happen. It isn't at all: I know what's happening. But a dog is a happy thing, and it will be happy for me for whatever time I've got left and as happy as things can be for my family when I've gone. ( *John Diamond*, pp. 255–6.)

## Section 2: The illness experience – the child

*Jenny Hynson*

This section will discuss the factors that influence the child's experience of illness in the palliative care setting. These are:

- the underlying condition
- developmental factors
- the ability of their parents and other caregivers to support them
- decisions made regarding their treatment.

## Life-limiting conditions encountered in pediatrics

The experience of illness is dependent on many variables, not least of which is the nature of the illness itself. In terms of the disease processes encountered, the patient population in pediatric palliative care is heterogeneous.[45–50] More than half of children who need palliative care have non-malignant conditions, and many of these have neuro-degenerative disorders, which cause a slow decline over months to years.

Congenital anomalies also account for a significant proportion of children who need palliative care. These can occur in isolation as fatal abnormalities of the central nervous system or heart, or as part of a constellation of abnormalities which together threaten the life of the child (e.g. trisomy 13 and 18). Some children are affected by disease processes which are very rare or unique. Occasionally, an exact diagnosis cannot be made. In such circumstances, prognosticating is extremely difficult and predictions can only be based on the observed progression in that particular child. It is in this context that parents and clinicians must make critical decisions on the child's behalf.

It is helpful to think of the conditions encountered in pediatric palliative care in terms of their course of progression. Four categories have been described:[49]

1. conditions for which curative treatment exists but fails in the particular child (e.g. malignant conditions), where there is often a clearer shift in the goal of care from curative to palliative
2. conditions in which intensive treatment can prolong and enhance life but premature death occurs (e.g. cystic fibrosis)
3. progressive conditions where no disease-modifying treatment exists and management is exclusively palliative (e.g. many neuro-degenerative conditions)
4. conditions where the underlying lesion is static but the complications are progressive and predispose the child to premature death (severe cerebral palsy is not in itself a progressive condition but the resultant musculoskeletal effects are, and lead to respiratory complications).

Of the malignant conditions that affect children, hematological malignancies and central nervous system tumors are the most frequently encountered. The former group is dominated by acute lymphoblastic leukemia, which now has an 80% cure rate.[50] The latter group is dominated by tumors of the posterior fossa, many of which still carry an extremely poor prognosis. Huge overall gains in survival rates for children with cancer have been made in the last 20 to 30 years, due mostly to carefully conducted clinical trials. Phase 1 trials to assess the safety, tolerability and efficacy of various agents continue to be important in pediatric oncology, but it can be difficult for parents and clinicians to decide on the place of such interventions in circumstances where the child's disease appears incurable.

It is important that parents are not forced to choose between ongoing attempts at cure and palliative care. Rather, the two can be combined successfully in a 'hope for the best, prepare for the worst' approach.[51,52] A high symptom burden among children in the terminal phase of malignant disease is well documented.[53-55] The most commonly encountered symptoms include pain, fatigue, dyspnea, anorexia, nausea, constipation and psychological symptoms such as anxiety. Depression is probably under-recognized in this group.

Neuro-degenerative conditions may progress in a range of ways, with variable time courses depending on the underlying disease process. These children are faced with the progressive loss of neurological function. For some, cognitive function is minimally affected and they are acutely aware of their increasing disability. For others, cognitive function deteriorates in parallel with physical impairment. Some of these conditions have their onset in infancy and are manifested by developmental delay and subsequent regression. Others are diagnosed later in childhood. Early signs of the condition may be cause for only minor parental concern but they herald the beginning of a slow and inexorable decline over months to years. Children in the advanced stages of neuro-degenerative disease face problems with communication, mobility and feeding.[56,57] They may also suffer from seizures, muscle spasm, irritability, constipation and pain related to musculoskeletal complications and gastro-oesophageal reflux.

Children in these circumstances are fully dependent on others for all their care needs. Parents generally provide this care as a natural extension of their parenting role, but it is a massive task involving regular turning, gastrostomy feeds, suctioning and the management of seizures, constipation and other complications. There are often multiple individuals and agencies involved in assisting families, as well as frequent hospital appointments and the presence of carers in the home. The need for home modifications and the various aids needed to safely care for the child may lead parents to feel that their home is becoming 'hospitalized'.[58]

Aspiration and chronic lung disease are frequent – and often fatal – complications. Children with such conditions are vulnerable to death, but prognosticating in these circumstances can be extremely difficult. They are faced with 'certain death at an unknown time'.[59] Children may have multiple episodes where death appears imminent. Miraculous recovery may engender a sense that the child is a 'fighter' or that the doctors have somehow 'got it wrong'. Parents may be reluctant to forgo life-sustaining measures in the face of such uncertainty. Indeed, death can ultimately come as a surprise despite the obvious vulnerability of the child.[47]

There is a range of conditions in which very active treatment can enhance and prolong life but premature death is likely if not certain. Cystic fibrosis and pulmonary hypertension are two examples. The possibility of organ transplantation in both scenarios means that the child, their family and the staff caring for them must balance dual goals. Simultaneously they must work towards transplant as well as facing the reality that the child may not survive the wait, the surgical procedure or the post-operative phase. Although many see these two goals as dichotomous, they need not be mutually exclusive. Children and families can be encouraged to retain hope while being supported around issues related to death and dying. Honest and open communication, careful decision-making and assistance to achieve the best possible quality of life are elements of palliative care that can be integrated into the overall management plan.[60]

## Development

Although adults continue to develop and change as they age, childhood is a period of rapid physical, emotional, psychological and spiritual growth. All of these dimensions affect a child's experience of illness, but the reverse is also true. Illness can delay a child's developmental progress, but the experience can also make a child wise beyond their years. In this way, the relationship between development and the illness experience is bi-directional, so that a child's developmental status is not a direct function of chronological age. There is a high degree of variability between individuals, and many of the conditions that affect children also cause neurological impairment and significant developmental delay. Developmental level influences the child's:

◗ understanding of death
◗ understanding of illness
◗ ability to communicate their concerns and symptoms
◗ capacity for decision-making.

### Understanding of death

A child's understanding of death is influenced by his or her developmental level, cognitive capacity and life experience.[66] A young child who has had a pet die, for example, may understand more about death than an older child who has had no similar experience. This is dependent, however, on how the experience is explained to the child. Most children learn to recognize when something is dead by the time they reach three years of age, but they may not be able to distinguish easily between death, separation and sleep. As children develop and experience life, their concept of death becomes progressively more mature. Seven sub-concepts are acquired during this process, and while there are set average ages of attainment (*see* Table 4.3), it is important to remember that there is considerable variability.[67] Further, illness or distress can cause developmental regression, leading a child to function at a less mature level (*see* Table 4.3).

**TABLE 4.3** Concepts required in the understanding of death, and the average age of attainment

| CONCEPT (AVERAGE AGE OF ONSET) | NATURE OF UNDERSTANDING OF THE CONCEPT |
|---|---|
| Separation (age 5) | The dead do not co-exist with the living. |
| Causality (age 6) | Death is caused by something, be it trauma, disease or old age. |
| Irreversibility (age 6) | A dead person can not 'come alive' again. |
| Non-functionality (age 6) | Bodily functions cease. |
| Universality (age 6) | All living things die. |
| Personal mortality (age 8) | 'I will die' |
| Insensitivity (age 8) | The dead can not feel fear or pain. |

In general, children younger than six years of age have not yet acquired the concept of irreversibility and may not understand that a dead person will not return. To them, death is a temporary state. The language used by adults at the time a person dies may be confusing in this context. For example, the statement, 'We lost Grandpa last night', might be met with a request that a search be organized. Many fairy tales and television shows reinforce the young child's understanding of death as a temporary state (e.g. Snow White died but returned to life, and Wile E. Coyote recovered from many terminal episodes).

Young children have a tendency to think 'magically'. Those who do not understand causality may believe they brought about the death of a loved person through their actions or wishes.[63] Children who do not see death as a part of the life cycle may see death as punishment for wrongdoing. Other children may need reassurance about the well-being of other members of the family.

At various points in their development, children may understand one sub-concept of death but not another. For example, a seven-year-old who understands that bodily functions like breathing and movement cease after a person dies may not necessarily appreciate that the person can not feel pain or fear. This may lead them to imagine someone they love being alone and immobile but frightened or distressed. Children may be able to understand the concept of universal mortality but not as it relates to them. These situations require careful management and it is helpful for families and those involved in caring for them to understand how children view death and what misconceptions they might have at various ages. More important, though, is an assessment of the individual child's level of understanding before conversations are had.

Young children often incorporate themes of death and dying into play. Parents may need reassurance that play is the child's way of making sense of their world and that it is normal for recent life experiences to be played out with toys or friends.

*Understanding of illness*

As with concepts of death, the way in which children understand illness is influenced by their developmental level, cognitive ability and the experience they have had of their own illness, as well as the observed experience of their peers. A child's level of understanding is also necessarily influenced by the information they receive from those around them. Information is gathered from parents, health professionals and fellow patients and pieced together to form a whole. This information comes in verbal and non-verbal forms, and children are very sensitive to discrepancies between the two. A child who is told that everything is fine but who sees their parents crying is quick to deduce that all is not well. Unfortunately, they may make incorrect assumptions about the reason for their parents' distress. These might include fears that their parents are experiencing problems in their relationship or even that that the child has done something to upset them.

It is known that children are very active in seeking information about their predicament. They listen keenly to the advice of more experienced patients on the ward or in the clinic waiting area, may eavesdrop on conversations between parents and staff and are very strategic in the way they ask questions.[64] In general, and in spite of the best efforts of others to try to protect them, sick children have a more sophisticated understanding of their illness than might be expected.

Children with malignancies have been described as progressing through five stages of understanding:

- Stage 1: I am seriously ill
- Stage 2: I am seriously ill but will get better
- Stage 3: I am always ill but will get better
- Stage 4: I am always ill and will not get better
- Stage 5: I am dying.

The fifth stage is characterized by a preoccupation with death in conversation and play, oppositional behaviour in relation to procedures and medication, and a reluctance to discuss events in the future.

Infants and toddlers understand illness in terms of the physical discomfort caused by symptoms and procedures, but perhaps more importantly as separation from important figures in their lives and the familiarity of the home environment. The impact of the diagnosis of life-limiting illness on parents is also felt by young children, who are acutely sensitive to changes in the emotional state of those closest to them.[65] Routines are often disrupted and parents may find it difficult to provide comfort and enforce boundaries when they are so distressed.

Although preschoolers have much in common with younger children, they have progressed to a developmental stage where their tendency to think magically may mean they view illness and painful procedures as punishment for wrongdoing.[66] They may also have a view of illness as contagious. Play becomes an important way of making sense of the world. School-aged children develop increasing independence and become more reliant on peers for support. They often have concerns about being seen as different. School represents a significant part of the child's life and is more than a place of learning: it is a center of social activity for the child and family and may provide a reassuring sense of normality and routine.

Adolescent patients have a greater capacity for abstract thinking and are more able to understand the implications of their condition and the various treatment options. They are therefore able to participate more actively in decision-making. They also have a more developed sense of the future and what it is they will lose through early death. Long-term relationships, child bearing and employment are all experiences the dying adolescent will miss. This can lead to an urgent need to live life as fully as possible by attending parties, drinking alcohol and engaging in sexual relationships. Young people may ignore the advice of parents and doctors to achieve these goals.

One of the developmental tasks of adolescence is to work towards autonomy and independence. The dependence created by illness is in direct conflict with this task and may cause frustration and distress.[67] The adolescent is also becoming more reliant on peers for support, and these important relationships may be disrupted by illness and hospitalization. Normal concerns about body image are exacerbated in young people whose illness causes physical changes such as weight loss, weight gain or disfigurement.

Although there is little known of the spiritual suffering of children with life-limiting conditions, it is important not to forget this dimension.[68] The development of illness affects the child's understanding of the world and his or her relationships with others.[69]

## References

1 Kaye P. *Breaking Bad News: a ten step approach*. EPL Publications: Northampton, UK; 1995.

2 Baile WF, Buckman R, Lenzi R, *et al.* SPIKES – a six-step protocol for delivering bad news: application to the patient with cancer. *Oncologist.* 2000; **5**: 302–11.

3 Pereira Gray D. Forty-seven minutes a year for the patient. *Br J Gen Pract.* 1998; **48**: 1816–17.

4 Seamark DA, Ryan M, Smallwood N, *et al.* Deaths from heart failure in general practice: implications for primary care. *Palliat Med.* 2002; **16**: 495–8.

5 Muntwyler J, Abetel G, Gruner C, *et al.* One year mortality among unrelated outpatients with heart failure. *Eur Heart J.* 2002; **23**: 1861–6.

6 Curtis JR, Wenrich MD, Carline JD, *et al.* Patients' perspectives on physician skill in end-of-life care: differences between patients with COPD, cancer and AIDS. *Chest.* 2002; **122**: 356–62.

7  Meredith C, Symonds P, Webster L, *et al*. Information needs of cancer patients in west Scotland: cross sectional survey of patients' views. *BMJ* 1996; **313**: 724–6.

8  Tierney W, Dexter P, Gramelspacher G, *et al*. The effects of discussion about advance directions on patients' satisfaction with primary care. *J Gen Intern Med*. 2001; **16**: 32–40.

9  Hammas B, Rooney B. Death and end-of-life planning in one Midwestern community. *Arch Intern Med*. 1998; **158**: 383–90.

10  Elkington H, White P, Higgs R, *et al*. GP's views of discussion of prognosis in severe COPD. *Family Pract*. 2001; **18**: 440–4.

11  Seamark DA, Blake SD, Seamark CJ, *et al*. Living with severe chronic obstructive pulmonary disease (COPD): perceptions of patients and their carers. *Palliat Med*. 2004; **18**: 619–25.

12  Fallowfield LJ, Jenkins VA, Beveridge HA. Truth may hurt but deceit hurts more: communication in palliative care. *Palliat Med*. 2002; **16**: 297–303.

13  Fallowfield L. Editorial: Participation of patients in decisions about treatment for cancer. *BMJ* 2001; **323**: 1144.

14  Diamond J. *C Because Cowards Get Cancer Too . . .* London: Random House; 2001.

15  Murray SA, Boyd K, Sheikh A. Palliative care in chronic illness. *BMJ* 2005; **330**: 611–12.

16  Lynn J. Serving patients who may die soon and their families: the role of hospice and other services. *JAMA* 2001: **285**: 925–32.

17  Halliwell J, Mulcahy P, Buetow S, *et al*. GP discussion of prognosis with patients with severe chronic obstructive pulmonary disease: a qualitative study. *Br J Gen Pract*. 2004; **54**: 904–8.

18  Murray SA, Boyd K, Sheikh A, *et al*. Developing primary palliative care. *BMJ* 2004; **329**: 1057–8.

19  Mitchell GK. How well do general practitioners deliver palliative care?: a systematic review. *Palliat Med*. 2002; **16**: 457–64.

20  McKinley RK, Stokes T, Exley C, *et al*. Care of people dying with malignant and cardiorespiratory disease in general practice. *Br J Gen Pract*. 2004; **54**: 909–13.

21  Gore JM, Brophy CJ, Greenstone MA. How well do we care for patients with end stage chronic obstructive pulmonary disease (COPD)?: a comparison of palliative care and quality of life in COPD and lung cancer. *Thorax*. 2000; **55**: 1000–6.

22  Hanratty B, Hibbert D, Mair F, *et al*. Doctors' perceptions of palliative care for heart failure: focus group study. *BMJ* 2002; **325**: 581–5.

23  Murray SA, Boyd K, Kendall M, *et al*. Dying of lung cancer or cardiac failure: prospective qualitative study of patients and their carers in the community. *BMJ* 2002; **325**: 929–33.

24  Pantilat SZ, Steimle AE. Palliative care for patients with heart failure. *JAMA* 2004; **291**: 2476–82.

25  Elkington H, White P, Addington-Hall J, *et al*. The last year of life of COPD: a qualitative study of symptoms and services. *Respir Med*. 2004; **98**: 439–45.

26  Jones I, Kirby A, Ormiston P, *et al*. The needs of patients dying of chronic obstructive pulmonary disease in the community. *Family Pract*. 2004; **21**: 310–13.

27  Addington-Hall J, McCarthy M. Regional study of care for the dying: methods and sample characteristics. *Palliat Med*. 1995; **9**: 27–35.

28  McCarthy M, Lay M, Addington-Hall J. Dying from heart disease. *J Roy Coll Physicians*. 1996; **30**: 325–8.

29 Lynn J, Teno JM, Phillips RS, *et al*. Perceptions of family members of the dying experience of older and seriously ill patients. *Ann Int Med*. 1997; **126**: 97–106.

30 Gibbs LME, Addington-Hall J, Gibbs JSR. Dying from heart failure: lessons from palliative care. *BMJ* 1998; **317**: 961–2.

31 Ellershaw J, Ward C. Clinical review: care of the dying patient: the last hours or days of life. *BMJ* 2003; **326**: 30–4.

32 Thomas K . *Caring for the Dying at Home: companions on the journey*. Oxford: Radcliffe Medical; 2003.

33 Higginson IJ, Astin P, Dolan S. Where do cancer patients die?: ten-year trends in the place of death of cancer patients in England. *Palliat Med*. 1998; **12**: 353–63.

34 Hinton J. Can home care maintain an acceptable quality of life for patients with terminal cancer and their relatives? *Palliat Med*. 1994; **8**: 183–96.

35 Murray SA, Kendall M, Boyd K, *et al*. Exploring the spiritual needs of people dying of lung cancer or heart failure: a prospective qualitative interview study of patients and their carers. *Palliat Med*. 2004; **18**: 39–45.

36 Grande GE, Barclay SIG, Todd CJ. Difficulty of symptom control and general practitioners' knowledge of patients' symptoms. *Palliat Med*. 1997; **11**: 399–406.

37 Higginson I, Sen-Gupta GJA. Place of care in advanced cancer. *J Palliat Med*. 2000; **3**: 287–300.

38 Hinton J. Which patients with terminal cancer are admitted from home care? *Palliat Med*. 1994; **8**: 197–210.

39 Seamark DA, Williams S, Hall M, *et al*. Palliative terminal cancer care in community hospitals and a hospice: a comparative study. *Br J Gen Pract*. 1998; **48**: 1312–16.

40 Seamark DA, Williams S, Hall M, *et al*. Dying from cancer in community hospitals or a hospice: closest lay carers' perceptions. *Br J Gen Pract*. 1998; **48**: 1317–21.

41 www.statistics.gov.uk/themehealth/DH1352002/DH1no35.pdf. Accessed 26.04.05.

42 Steinhauser KE, Clipp EC, McNeilly M, *et al*. In search of a good death: observations of patients, families and providers. *Ann Int Med*. 2000; **132**: 825–32.

43 Stevenson J, Abernethy AP, Miller C, *et al*. Managing co-morbidities in patients at the end of life. *BMJ* 2004; **329**: 909–12.

44 Thorne CP, Seamark DA, Lawrence C, *et al*. The influence of general practitioner community hospitals on the place of death of cancer patients. *Palliat Med*. 1994; **8**: 122–8.

45 Hynson J, Sawyer S. Paediatric palliative care: distinctive needs and emerging issues. *J Paed Child Health*. 2001; **37**: 323–5.

46 Feudtner CD, Zimmerman FJ, Muldoon JH, *et al*. Characteristics of deaths occurring in children's hospitals: implications for supportive care services. *Pediatrics*. 2002; **109**: 887–93.

47 Jones R, Trenholme A, Horsburgh M, *et al*. The need for paediatric palliative care in New Zealand. *NZ Med J*. 2002; **115**(1163): 198.

48 Hutchinson F, King N, Hain R. Terminal care in paediatrics: where we are now. *Postgrad Med J*. 2003; **79**: 566–8.

49 Goldman A. ABC of palliative care: special problems of children. *BMJ* 1998; **316**: 49–52.

50 Ziegler D, Dalla Pozza L, Waters K, *et al*. Advances in childhood leukaemia: successful clinical-trials research leads to individualised therapy. *MJA*. 2005; **182**: 78–81.

51 Ulrich C, Grady C, Wendler D. Palliative care: a supportive adjunct to pediatric phase 1 clinical trials for anticancer agents. *Pediatrics.* 2004; **114**: 852–5.

52 Back A, Arnold R, Quill T. Hope for the best, and prepare for the worst. *Ann Intern Med.* 2003; **138**: 439–43.

53 Wolfe J, Grier H, Klar N, *et al.* Symptoms and suffering at the end of life in children with cancer. *N Engl J Med.* 2000; **342**: 326–33.

54 Collins J, Byrnes M, Dunkel I, *et al.* The measurement of symptoms in children with cancer. *J Pain Symptom Manage.* 2000; **19**: 363–77

55 Drake R, Frost J, Collins J. The symptoms of dying children. *J Pain Symptom Manage.* 2003; **26**: 594–603.

56 Hunt A, Burne R. Medical and nursing problems of children with neurodegenerative disease. *Palliat Med.* 1995; **9**: 19–26.

57 Lenton S, Stallard P, Mastroyannopoulou K. Prevalence and morbidity associated with non-malignant, life-threatening conditions in childhood. *Child Care Health Dev.* 2001; **27**: 389–98.

58 Wray D, Wray S. Andrew: a journey – a parents' perspective. *Child Care Health Dev.* 2004; **30**: 201–2.

59 Steele R. Trajectory of certain death at an unknown time: children with neurodegenerative life-threatening illnesses. *Can J Nurs Research.* 2000; **32**: 49–67.

60 Robinson W, Ravilly S, Berde C, *et al.* End-of-life care in cystic fibrosis. *Pediatrics.* 1997; **100**: 205–9.

61 Reilly T, Hazazi J, Bond L. Children's conceptions of death and personal mortality. *J Ped Psychol.* 1983; **8**: 21–31.

62 Kenyon B. Current research in children's conceptions of death: a critical review. *Omega.* 2001; **43**: 63–91.

63 Kane B. Children's concepts of death. *J Genet Psychol.* 1979; **134**: 141–53.

64 Bluebond-Langner, M. *The Private Worlds of Dying Children.* Princeton, N.J.: Princeton University Press; 1978.

65 Barakat L, Sills R, LaBagnara S. Management of fatal illness and death in children or their parents. *Ped Rev.* 1995; **16**: 419–23.

66 Brewster A. Chronically ill hospitalized children's concepts of their illness. *Pediatrics.* 1982; **69**: 355–62.

67 Carr-Gregg M, Sawyer S, Clarke C, *et al.* Caring for the terminally ill adolescent. *Med J Aust.* 1997; **166**: 255–8.

68 Davies B, Brenner P, Orloff S, *et al.* Addressing spirituality in pediatric hospice and palliative care. *J Palliat Care.* 2002; **18**: 59–67.

69 Attig T. Beyond pain: the existential suffering of children. *J Palliat Care.* 1996; **12**: 20–3.

## Resources and websites

**Canadian Cancer Society**

This website has a wide range of information for patients, primary carers and friends. The information is written for a lay person. There are pages with high-quality evidence for those who want to delve more deeply into the subject.

www.cancer.ca

**CancerBACUP** is Europe's leading cancer information service, with up-to-date cancer information, practical advice and support for cancer patients, their families and carers.
www.cancerbacup.org.uk

### Cancer Council Australia

This site has a page called 'Common questions about cancer', which provides written information about a wide range of cancer questions written for lay people, as well as a wide array of information for clinicians.
www.cancer.org.au

### Caresearch

This Australian website has a section with information for patients, carers, family and friends. It is also a repository of research-based tools for clinicians, and a library of grey literature around palliative care.
www.caresearch.com.au

**DIPEx** is a registered UK charity with an ongoing program of collecting personal experiences of health and illness. Researchers have identified patients and their carers through primary care and specialist services, and have undertaken in-depth interviews, which are audiotaped and video-recorded. The site covers cancers, heart disease, mental health, neurological conditions, screening programs, chronic illness and teenage health and pregnancy. The patient, carer or health professional can watch or read the interviews and find reliable information on treatment choices and where to find support. For those with life-threatening illnesses, there are detailed accounts of receiving bad news, finding information, treatment decisions and symptoms, facing death, religion, faith and philosophy. The site is being added to constantly.
www.dipex.org

**Macmillan Cancer Relief** is involved in providing help to people living with cancer. It also facilitates health professionals in palliative care roles and has a research and development role.
www.macmillan.org.uk

### Marie Curie Cancer Care

This UK charity provides an information service and has hospices and people to help cancer patients in the community. It is also involved in research.
www.mariecurie.org.uk

### National Cancer Institute, USA

This site contains a vast array of information on cancer, much of it in the form of fact sheets about specific diseases and treatments. Most lay information is in the cancer topics section.
http://www.cancer.gov/cancertopics

### National Electronic Library of Health

This is an NHS initiative for patients and health professionals aimed at providing up-to-date information and resources for good care.
www.nelh.nhs.uk

**People Living with Cancer**
A site from the USA developed by the American Society of Clinical Oncology, this has a very patient-friendly layout. Advice and information about palliative care are in the section on diagnosis and treatment.
www.plwc.org

# CHAPTER 5

# Understanding the whole person: life-limiting illness across the life cycle

*GEOFFREY MITCHELL, JUDITH MURRAY, JENNY HYNSON*

## Introduction

Previous chapters have examined disease processes in life-limiting conditions and how they have affected the sufferer. However, there is also an impact on the person's relationship with the external world, which is profound for all involved. Following on from the previous chapter, we will show how much of the impact on the ill person's interactions with others relates to their perception of, and response to, losses occurring at this critical time. How healthcare professionals can respond to these losses is also discussed.

The previous chapter approached the issue from the perspective of critical points in the illness trajectory. This chapter examines the proximal context by offering an approach to the end of life based on the individual's response to loss and forced change. It then examines how these responses affect external relationships, and how those people close to the affected person might respond in return.

Miller and Omarzu[1] define loss as follows:

> Loss is produced by an event which is perceived to be negative by the individual involved and results in long-term changes to one's social situations, relationships, or cognitions. (p. 12)

Life-limiting illness introduces loss into the life of a person and those close to him or her. Grief, broadly defined as the reaction to loss, then permeates their lives.

Being ill changes many aspects of a person's life. Multiple losses impact simultaneously, constituting the experience of illness. As a result, the grief response in illness is more complex than grieving the loss of health alone, and each person associated with the ill person will also experience losses. Practitioners need to be ready to respond to each individual's personal loss.

There are many factors that will affect the process of grieving, an important one being the point of the life cycle at which the illness becomes part of a person's experience. This chapter will also consider different points in the life cycle, the impact of illness on patients of different ages, their loved ones and carers. Jenny Hynson has provided the section of this chapter devoted to the unique problems encountered when the dying person is a child or adolescent.

## Section 1: A framework for considering life-limiting illness across the life cycle
*Judith Murray and Geoffrey Mitchell*

### Understanding responses to loss
Both the person suffering a life-limiting illness and those close to the individual are affected by losses.

### *The whole person*
There are several dimensions to the human experience, including a person's physical health and well-being, personality traits, learned psychological responses to stress and pressure, and spiritual beliefs. A well person integrates these into a unified whole. When illness strikes, the person remains the same whole person, yet somehow everything is changed. The very characteristics that make humans unique lead to unpleasant experiences over and above the sickness.

For a start, we have *recall* – we remember what it was like to be healthy. We may have *regret* that this is not the case now, and wish for a return to health. We *anticipate* what will happen in the future. When the future includes imminent death, our *imagination* can lead to despair. Well people can *plan* for the future, and have hopes and aspirations. When the hoped-for future is denied by life-limiting illness, what then? Grief – the response to losses – can produce distressing physical, psychological, behavioural, social and spiritual effects (*see* Table 5.1) As a result, teasing out the contributions of physical illness and grief to the patient's presentation can be challenging.

**TABLE 5.1** Manifestations of grief

| PHYSICAL | PSYCHOLOGICAL/EMOTIONAL | BEHAVIORAL | SOCIAL | SPIRITUAL |
|---|---|---|---|---|
| Palpitations | Moodiness | Poor concentration | Intentional social isolation | Intense spiritual search |
| Headaches | Irritability | Forgetfulness | Relationship tensions | Rejection of previous beliefs and practices |
| Body aches | Depressed mood | Slowness of thinking and decision-making | Reluctance to leave home | Anger at God |
| Stiffness | Apathy | Difficulty expressing oneself verbally | Frequent arguments, family difficulties | Fear of judgement |
| Weakness | Guilt | Disorientation | Increase in use of alcohol, tobacco and other drugs | Doubts and modification of prior beliefs |
| Fatigue | Restlessness, excitability | Overactivity | Fear of being alone | Questions meaning of life |
| Changes in eating patterns | Sadness, crying | Inability to carry out even the most minor tasks | Shortness with the daily concerns of others | Strict adherence to religious practices |
| Faintness | Feeling lost, isolated, abandoned | Difficulty in organizing daily tasks | Drifting away to own thoughts during conversation | |
| Sighing | Recurrent dreams | Eating more or less | Seeking out those in similar circumstances | |
| Trouble breathing | Insomnia | Loss of work efficiency | Rejection of those in similar circumstances | |
| Rapid shallow breathing | Night waking | Easily startled | | |
| Numbness | Expressions of frustration | | | |
| Tingling or heaviness in arms or legs | Anxiety | | | |
| Susceptibility to colds | Fears, worry | | | |
| 'Allergies' | Feeling overwhelmed, powerless | | | |
| Chills | Hopelessness | | | |
| Nausea | Guilt | | | |
| Upset stomach | Blaming | | | |
| Diarrhea | Numbness | | | |
| Constipation | Shock | | | |
| Tremors of hands, lips etc. | Confusion | | | |
| Sleep disturbances | Inability to feel | | | |
| Faintness | Loss of interest in sex | | | |
| Dizziness | | | | |
| Sensation of 'lump in throat' | | | | |
| Lack of co-ordination | | | | |

## Grieving, suffering and mourning

In the palliative care setting there are myriad losses. Some of these are mentioned in Table 5.2. Sometimes the losses are obvious, such as loss of a normal physical function. Others are losses of potential, of dignity, of independence.

Mourning is the *emotion* associated with loss, and grieving is the *process* of adjusting to the loss. The degree of *suffering* experienced reflects the size of the gap between what is and what is desired. Suffering is a part of grief. MacIntosh defines suffering as 'a consequence of self-awareness, and occurs when a person's current state fails to match a state he or she is able to accept'.[2]

Mourning occurs to differing degrees in different people. The professional needs to identify which losses are important, and in what way, in order to help the sufferers to deal with them appropriately. A loss that may appear trivial to the observer may be catastrophic to the sufferer: misunderstandings may arise. Hence the health professional must assess the importance of each loss. Can something be done to ameliorate the losses? Can the practitioner prioritize his or her actions in line with the patient's perceived losses?

## Suffering through looking back

For some, the response to loss is to reflect on the past, to what the situation was before the loss. The effect of this is as if the loss event has placed a transparent glass wall between the past and the present. The individual may look back at the situation that existed before but may not return. Some patients have great difficulty shifting their gaze from the view back through the glass, suffering greatly because the return journey is not possible. There is no thought to move forward. This manifests itself as an abnormal grief reaction, which can cause impairment for years.

## Example

Dr Tony's next patient is Phyllis B. These visits are always difficult. Phyllis's consultations always come back to the same thing: she misses her husband David terribly.

David presented with persistent upper abdominal discomfort several months before his pancreatic carcinoma was diagnosed. He died nine months after an exploratory laparotomy found the cancer, two years ago. Phyllis adored David. They were more than husband and wife: they were the best of friends. It was David who looked after the finances, the home maintenance, and took all the decisions about what they would do next. The two of them looked forward to 'doing the big lap' – circumnavigating Australia in a motor home. All that is gone, and she is completely lost.

Phyllis's monologues range from her gambling-addicted son Peter, to the

**TABLE 5.2** Losses associated with life-limiting illness

**Loss of:**

- the perceived future, or any future if the illness is terminal
- life is contemplated, which is distressing both when the person may not fully understand what that means (e.g. a young child) *and* for an adult well aware of what that means
- normal social interactions with others due to:
  - life revolving around the illness and treatments
  - feeling different to peers and uncomfortable in their presence
  - being confined to home
- time and recreation (to time-consuming and often unpleasant treatments or care procedures)
- enjoyment of activities previously enjoyed, or that provided a diversion
- the ability to distract thoughts away from the situation and see life the way others do
- companionship – there is a sense of loneliness when putting on a 'brave' face
- membership of the peer group when away from work or school for long periods of time
- social support when a stigmatized illness is perceived as being at least partially self-inflicted
- being a normal part of the family when hospitalized and not participating in everyday home life
- relationships with caregivers and other family members
- childhood experiences for an ill child
- dignity and privacy during treatment
- control of body functions
- independence
- freedom, where caregivers become over-protective or a dependency relationship becomes established
- trust, if a person senses things are being hidden from him or her
- security, with the death of other patients with whom the patient may have shared the hospital experience
- self-esteem, if body changes make the person 'stand out in the crowd' or are particularly offensive, such as an odorous tumor
- self-esteem, when the disease forces even relatively simple tasks to be done by others
- relationships and support, due to changes in professional staff from transfers or moving into a different part of the health system
- 'their place', such as their own room and bed etc. when hospitalized
- security, if the strain of the illness leads to stresses between themselves and caregivers, or between caregivers.

motor home sitting idle in the backyard, to her struggles with financial decisions, and always back to how much she misses her best friend. 'I feel like someone has cut off my right arm!' she says, through her tears.

Dr Tony can hardly get a word in edgeways. He just listens. Phyllis decides when the consultation has finished, and always thanks Dr Tony for being so understanding and helping so much. Bemused, Dr Tony asks himself what he has really done for Phyllis this time, and the numerous times before, as he ushers the next patient into the room.

Phyllis clearly put her life on hold when David died. She is rooted firmly on the wrong side of the glass wall, looking back at what has been lost. The problem for Dr Tony is what to do.

## The importance of the person's story

A patient's response to their circumstances may be better understood by understanding those elements of their story most likely to be felt as losses. These can be identified with a few key questions (*see* Table 5.3).

**TABLE 5.3** Key questions to elucidate the patient's story

| | |
|---|---|
| **What past events define this person?** | Schooling |
| | Employment history |
| | Consuming hobbies or passions |
| | A single defining moment like a motor vehicle accident |
| **What are the most important relationships in this person's life (these can be positive or negative influences)?** | Life partner, children or close relatives |
| | People from the past (e.g. teachers, school friends) |
| | Workmates |
| | Friends in sporting clubs or church |
| **What are the person's spiritual beliefs? How important are they to him or her?** | These can be an enormous comfort and source of strength, but they can also be a major stumbling block to understanding the illness and treatments offered |
| **Are there relevant cultural issues?** | Attitudes to illness and prognosis disclosure |
| | Decision-making: autonomy versus involvement of family members |
| | Understanding of death and the afterlife |
| **Prior experience or observations of people being ill?** | Past observations of persons with severe illness |
| | Relevance of past observations to current observations |
| | These can be an enormous comfort and source of strength, but they can also be a major stumbling block to understanding the illness and treatments offered |
| **What are the patient's greatest fears or regrets?** | Unfulfilled ambitions |
| | Future care of young children or older dependants |
| | Threatened financial security |
| | Going to heaven or hell |

## Different responses to loss

### Hope

How can hope be found in the face of increasing degeneration, incessant pain, and impending death? Hope differs from optimism in that it is grounded in reality.[3] Consequently, caring that facilitates hope must include an exploration of the situation as it really is for the suffering person. Carers will recognize that hope for a particular goal (e.g. to find a cure) differs from a more generic hope (e.g. that there is a future beyond death), best described as an 'openness of the spirit'. It may be necessary for those caring for an ill person to be prepared to address both types of hope or hopelessness.


## Chronic sorrow

In many situations of long-term illness, the trajectory and endpoint are not well defined. New challenges and losses constantly emerge. For example, people diagnosed with motor neurone disease will grieve at the time of diagnosis. However, the grief intensifies as they begin to gain an awareness of the conse-quences of the illness, become more and more dependent on others, and feel the injustice of not having the future they had hoped for.[4] Similarly, carers feel ongoing pain as the person's ability to live independently becomes compromised or their personality changes. Many people feel overwhelmed by the powerlessness of their situation. The long-term sadness that accompanies such ongoing losses was first termed *chronic sorrow* by Olshansky[5] in his study of parents whose children were confronted with a disability.

Teel has described episodes or cycles of sadness in chronic sorrow, during which the disparity between the world as they would like it to be and reality is more deeply felt.[6] During these times, hope can be very difficult to find. These more emotionally taxing episodes within chronic sorrow are usually time-limited, with periods of relative neutrality, satisfaction and happiness. However, some of the sadness always remains and can vary in intensity between situations and persons. As time goes on, and the person becomes more incapacitated, there may be longer periods where this more neutral relationship with the illness cannot be maintained. The sadness may progress and intensify years after the initial diagnosis and loss.[7]

When the patient is in a down time practitioners should avoid discussing concrete actions that may ameliorate the emotional response. The act of listening, and validating their sense of powerlessness, can alone be therapeutic.[8] When the sadness is less conspicuous, the person is better able to entertain more practical and cognitive discussions of coping. Practitioners are less likely to misinterpret the reactions of patients and families to a long-term illness if they recognize the fluctuating pattern of affective responses as chronic sorrow. At these low ebbs, the patient or family may need extra support to deal with what they may feel are insurmountable challenges.

At these times a diagnosis of depression may be considered. The same person in a more neutral part of the cycle will appear to be coping well, so caution in making such a diagnosis is warranted.[7] Depression is characterized by a pervasive loss of enjoyment and motivation, which can lead to an inability to function in daily life, while chronic sorrow does not significantly affect daily functioning. In fact, carers enduring chronic sorrow commonly show extraordinary efforts in the care of the ill person, as well as performing within other areas of their lives.

## Depression and anxiety

While essentially different, chronic sorrow and depression may be related. If each of the cumulative losses of progressive illness is not mourned, a depressive state may develop. Depression and chronic sorrow can co-exist.[9]

For some patients, theories proposing that depression is the result of learned helplessness,[10] hopelessness,[11] or the result of feeling trapped[12] may be relevant in understanding how their chronic sorrow may devolve into clinical depression. Coping resources can become depleted and previously employed strategies less effective when constantly facing serious illness and impending death. The sense of being 'trapped' may sap emotional, social and spiritual strength just as the disease saps physical strength.

The result is an intense response which, while debilitating, can respond to counselling techniques. Drug therapy may not be required. By contrast, patients with a biologically mediated depression can display an almost psychotic belief that circumstances are irretrievable, and they will often require drug therapy. Counseling alone is less likely to bring about complete relief.

Both depression and anxiety are commonly found among those affected by serious illness.[13,14] As a result, the use of psychoactive drugs is common in chronic illness and palliative care settings. Depression may affect the progress of the illness.[15] There is an overlap between the symptoms of chronic medical illness, the side-effects of medication, and the symptoms of depression,[16] and teasing out the contribution of each can be challenging. Altering a medication and/or improving symptom control may be the key to relieving disconcerting emotional responses.

## Suicide and euthanasia

In an uncomfortable article, Humphrey[17] argues that suicide can be a rational option taken by the elderly, and perhaps also by the ill. Suicide can be seen as a logical means of ending suffering when the end is in sight anyway. Others just become tired of living with constant pain and uncertainty. They can come to see suicide as a way of retaining control in an uncontrollable situation. Some may see suicide as a means of removing the burden of their illness from their family.[18]

## Example

George was a meticulous 73-year-old man with mesothelioma. The condition caused severe pain, which took much effort to control. In spite of this, George maintained a degree of activity, with daily walks to the shop to get the paper. His family loved him dearly, and wanted the very best for him. They insisted on preparing the home for the difficult days ahead. In spite of concerns expressed by Dr Sophia that they were thinking of this too soon, they arranged for an occupational therapist to measure up the house for hand rails and an invalid bath. The day after this visit George's mood took a nose dive. Several days later he quietly tidied the house, went to his workshop and hung himself. It appears he finally realized what was ahead for himself and his family, and decided to end it all to save his family the distress of looking after an invalid.

The issues of euthanasia and physician-assisted suicide are real for practitioners in a palliative care setting, compared to the largely academic argument that often ensues around this issue in the wider community. Euthanasia cases in palliative care are no longer interesting clinical curiosities. Most GPs can report making medical decisions that would hasten death, and one-third made decisions knowingly hastening death. One 20th of participants in a New Zealand survey had deliberately induced death in the last 12 months.[19] In Holland, requests for euthanasia are made at the rate of 2.6 per 10 000 population per annum.[20]

## How healthcare professionals can ease the struggle

Practitioners can often help to ease the difficulties of patients facing serious illness. The most important support practitioners can give may not be to exercise their professional skills, but their humanity. Practitioners can offer comfort for the fear, confusion and disappointments a life-limiting illness brings. They recognize and respect the grasping for hope and the existential pain of dying. This sort of care is of a different quality to that offered with a 'professional as expert' approach.

### Maximize safety and security

Illness robs people of a sense of mastery over their world and their future. To counter feelings of insecurity, the practitioner can offer patients support to feel 'more safe' in their uncertain world. Insecurity may be felt across all areas of life, so many disciplines may need to be involved in an attempt to restore safety (*see* Table 5.4)

While practitioners may strive to restore safety and security, this may not always be completely possible. The best that can be achieved may be to provide support to patients and carers distressed by the instability of the world that is.

**TABLE 5.4** Ways of enhancing a patient's sense of safety

Ensure adequacy of pain and other symptom control – complete pain relief may come at an unacceptable cost to the patient (e.g. drowsiness from narcotics).

Ease emotional distress:

■ identify the issues causing most distress
■ identify the presence of chronic sorrow and its attendant cyclical worsening
■ identify depression or anxiety, or exacerbations of previous mental health problems
■ identify aspects, activities or relationships that give hope
■ give permission to express distress.

Validate or challenge the person's view of his or her illness, including:

■ its causation
■ its meaning
■ the person's approach to the thought of dying.

Identify and address relationship difficulties, including:

■ family and friends
■ carers (both non-professional and professional)
■ whether professional caregivers are constant or changing (e.g. through transfers).

Assess the primary caregiver:

■ Has the primary caregiver accepted this role willingly?
■ Does the caregiver feel distressed by the burden of care?
■ Does caregiving change the relationship between carer and patient?

Recognize strains related to the illness trajectory, including:

■ repeated crises, which heighten prognostic uncertainty for the ill person and carers
■ patient and carers anticipating the end repeatedly.

Organizational issues, including:

■ whether appointments are timely and reliable
■ shared record keeping and communication
■ avoiding the patient repeating the story
■ identifying the leader of the care team (make this an overt choice, not one by default)
■ whether respite is available to carers, and the care is appropriate
■ identifying available community support, and utilising it
■ ascertaining whether ill people from rural and remote communities can be cared for in their community, and if not, how this disruption can be minimized
■ finding out what state financial assistance is available
■ minimizing financial strains – overt (e.g. drug selection) and covert (e.g. transport, parking, laundry).

## Help the patient move on

Having found themselves on the wrong side of the barrier that separates the 'world that is' from 'the world that was', the person ideally has to forge a new means of living that accounts for the new reality. This usually means reassessing his or her goals for living, and concentrating on those activities and relationships that have the greatest importance.

Consider the things that define the essence of the person and must be protected. These are elements fundamental to the individual, as opposed to the many others that are peripheral. Fundamental things might include the family and the patient's role in it. Illness may challenge personal spiritual beliefs, which may go through a process of transition and will have a key role in determining the person's response to the situation.

When the core set of interests and personal icons has been identified, the next thing is to help the person define what actions are possible to maintain them. Things that are peripheral can be released with less impact. It should be possible to formulate responses that allow the patients – and carers – to move on.

## Example

Phyllis is stuck on the wrong side of the barrier, looking back at the wonderful marriage she experienced with David. Eventually, Dr Tony manages to steer the conversation to the future. What are the things that are most important to Phyllis's life?

Phyllis has always wanted to be independent and not reliant on her family once the boys grew up. The motor-home lifestyle was really a manifestation of this desire. Phyllis is encouraged to consider what she can do to achieve this. She eventually decides that a move to a seaside city about two hours from her home would be the best for her. In fact she and David rented in this location for some months before the fateful cancer diagnosis changed everything.

Some time later she arrives at Dr Tony's surgery having sold her flat, and asks for the names of doctors in the seaside town. With his full blessing she departs shortly after. There are occasional trips back to see Dr Tony. She is very happy, and has made good connections with fellow residents in her new location. It takes a year for Phyllis to gather enough confidence in her new doctor at the coast not to have to make the four-hour round trip to see Dr Tony. This is three years after David's death.

Dr Tony has shown patience and persistence, slowly planting the idea of a new beginning in Phyllis's mind. In her own time she makes the decision, and life in this new phase begins in earnest.

### Helping the patient to finish with no regrets

Everyone wants to believe that they have passed on something of value to the next generation before he or she dies.[21] It is important to look back and believe one has led a purposeful life.[22] Not to feel like this can lead to distress in the last days.

The quality of interpersonal interactions is also important in determining the level of distress and remaining quality of life.[23–25] For surviving relatives, problems in the relationship may be associated with complicated grieving,[26,27] so it is helpful for the practitioner to help resolve issues that may lead to regrets for both themselves and the carers. Such issues include sorting out problematic family relationships, putting financial or spiritual affairs in order, completing a long-held dream or project, living long enough to be part of a significant family event, being able to find value in the life lived, or facing death in a way that will make the person feel proud.

### Example

Colin is driving his wife Marge mad. He has started to take over the running of the house. He has upgraded all the household goods, tidied the shed, renewed the car insurance, and drilled poor Marge on how to pay bills and keep the gutters clear. He demonstrates a desperate desire to get everything organized before the time comes when he is unable to 'pull his weight'.

Colin has a brain tumor, which has manifested itself almost immediately after retirement from a life in the police force. He attained the rank of Senior Sergeant, in charge of a regional station. Clearly a man in control, he found himself plunged into a situation where his life was out of control. Responding in the only way he knew how, Colin took charge of those things he could.

But there is something else in his desperation. When asked by Dr Sophia, 'What are you most frightened of?', the reply is that he is not certain that he will be accepted into heaven. He has lapsed into intermittent interest in his Presbyterian heritage and upbringing and has not taken Communion in years, and expresses fear that he will not 'make the grade' based on his life to date. Making contact with the local Presbyterian minister leads to regular visits to the home, talks about this life and the next, and the resumption of regular Communion. Colin becomes far more like his old self, and Marge can finally relax.

The following sections examine the issue of proximal context – what having a life-limiting illness does to the people caring for the person, and how the person with the illness responds to those closest to him or her. Because these issues differ as a person goes through the life cycle, the responses of children and adolescents, and then adults, are examined in detail.

# Section 2: Children and adolescents
*Jenny Hynson*

## Parental responses to caring for a child with life-limiting illness

It is expected that, to the best of their ability, parents will protect their children from injury, disease and death. The death of a child strikes at the very heart of what it means to be a parent, and amid the anticipated feelings of grief and sadness are feelings of guilt and failure. The grief parents experience is known to be more severe, prolonged and at greater risk of complication than any other form of grief.[28–30] There is even evidence to suggest that the mortality rate among bereaved parents is increased, especially among mothers who suffer the sudden or unexpected loss of their child.[31]

Factors associated with better outcomes among bereaved parents include:

▶ ongoing access to a source of emotional support[32]
▶ a life view that allows the parent to keep the diagnosis in perspective so that day-to-day family functioning can be maintained[32]
▶ accepting that some questions will never be resolved[32]
▶ an open communication style within the family that includes providing the sick child with information about the illness and its prognosis[32]
▶ caring for the child at home.

## Parental responses to the diagnosis of a life-limiting illness

Shock, disbelief and anger are common reactions to the diagnosis of fatal illness in a child.[33] Parents may look for some act or omission that may have caused the child's condition. This is often complicated by the fact that it often takes some time for the diagnosis to be made, and some parents may feel they should have been more aggressive in pursuing their concerns. Feelings of guilt are heightened in circumstances where the condition is inherited, and there may be tension in the family as blame is assigned to one or other parent.

Parents experience anticipatory grief from the time their child's condition is diagnosed. In addition to the death that will ultimately occur, parents must adjust to a series of other losses as the child progresses from well to ill, able to disabled. Parents may also experience a loss of control, privacy, income, employment and freedom.[34–36] It can become enormously difficult to plan even the simplest outing. At a more fundamental level, the diagnosis of fatal illness in a child is a threat to long-held assumptions about the natural order of things. These might include the assumption that children outlive their parents, or that life is fair and just.

## Learning to cope

Parents of children with life-threatening illnesses are thrown into an unfamiliar world. In addition to learning about their child's illness and its treatment, they must learn to negotiate a complex service system. There are also the physical requirements of caring for a dependent child. For most parents, taking their child home becomes a priority.[33] In the face of circumstances where they are unable to protect their child from disease and death, many feel this is something they can do – a wish they can fulfil.[37]

Some parents will learn complex nursing tasks to achieve this goal. These might include administering subcutaneous medication, replacing nasogastric tubes and operating ventilators. Internal conflict may be generated by attempts to combine the role of parent and nurse. Parents who must care for their children over many years are at risk of physical and emotional exhaustion.[38] It is not unusual for parents to harbor a secret wish that it would all end for the sake of the child and family. Considerable guilt may be associated with such thoughts, and it can be reassuring for parents to know they are not alone in experiencing them.

Parents generally regard caring for their dying child at home as a positive thing.[39–41] While children are smaller than adults and caring for them in sickness is a natural extension of the parenting role, the enormousness of this task cannot be overstated. Watching one's child die goes against all that is instinctive to a parent. There are also often long vigils at the child's bedside, physical tasks involved in providing care, and the emotional distress of family and friends.[42,43] They may be worried about their ability to keep the child comfortable and the accessibility and responsiveness of the service system. Young parents have often not seen a person die and there may be intense anxiety around the dying process and managing a dead body.

## Example

Carl is eight years old and has adrenoleucodystrophy. He lives at home with his mother and his sister aged 10. His parents have separated but his father visits frequently. Carl has limited movement and cannot communicate. His current problems include severe pain on transfer as a result of a subluxed hip, constipation, seizures, and frequent respiratory infections, which require hospitalization and sometimes ventilation. He is fed via a gastrostomy.

Carl is totally dependent and his mother is attending to him around the clock, turning him, feeding him, bathing him and administering medications. She can access only four hours of respite care each week and is feeling increasingly tired. She is taking antidepressants. During the last admission to hospital, Carl's pediatrician raised the question of whether Carl should be admitted to the Intensive Care Unit next time he suffered a respiratory infection. Carl's father became angry and stormed out of the meeting saying that the hospital was discriminating against his son on the grounds of disability. Carl's mother, on the other hand, could see that the interventions associated with ICU were intrusive, burdensome and unlikely to benefit Carl given his poor overall prognosis. She has accepted the assistance of a community-based palliative care team.

Parents may cling to the hope that their child will be cured or that a miracle will occur.[34] Even parents who seem able to discuss their child's prognosis openly, and accept support and even plan for the time of death, may harbor a secret hope that the child will survive. This may be a strategy that enables parents to cope with each day. It does not necessarily require 'breaking down' unless it is affecting the child's quality of life and care.

The complexity of the child's condition and frequent hospital admissions may cause families to rely on health professionals for emotional and social support to the exclusion of family and friends.[34] This may result in feelings of isolation when the child dies and parents find themselves disconnected from their usual support structure.

### After the death

Central to an understanding of the grief parents experience is the notion that parental feelings of protectiveness and attachment do not die with the child. For this reason it may take some time for parents to feel they can leave their child's body. It is also usual for parents to maintain an active connection with the child through possessions, rituals and creative endeavors such as writing and art. A number of parents continue to speak to the deceased child and some have an ongoing sense of the child's presence. These 'continuing bonds' can provide considerable comfort to the grieving parent.[44]

There may be gender differences in the way parents manage.[34] Mothers may prefer to talk about their experiences and feelings with others. Fathers may be less expressive, preferring to focus on practical issues. Fathers often describe feelings of helplessness.[33]

The travails of parents who must endure the illness and death of their child are well documented, but even in the face of such anguish some are able to describe positive aspects of their experience.[45-47] These include:

- an opportunity to say and do things with their child that others without the same pressure of time may never have
- experiencing the kindness of others and the opportunity to meet people they may not otherwise have encountered
- personal growth and the discovery or development of skills and attributes they would never have imagined.

## How professionals can respond to the dying child
### Communication

Of critical importance to the child is their ability to receive information that is appropriate to their level of development and their capacity to share their fears, hopes and wishes with those best able to support them (*see* Chapter 4, pp. 69–72). Parents often feel an instinctive need to 'protect' their child from the reality of what is happening. In some circumstances this is appropriate, but more often harm can be done by allowing the child to be alone with their concerns.[48] Studies have shown that even when parents are certain that their child 'knows' very little about the prognosis, the child is very aware of the possibility or probability of death. Just as parents try to protect children, children try to protect parents.[49] The fact that the issue is not discussed by the other party leads to the assumption that they are blissfully unaware of what is happening.

Children who do not have the opportunity to share their concerns are at risk of feeling isolated and anxious.[49] This is not to say that all children should be told bluntly, and without regard for their individual needs, the harsh facts of their situation. Children do not necessarily need to know all about their illness, and it is often possible to reassure and comfort them once their specific concerns are solicited and understood.

They are also likely to harbor distressing misconceptions.[50] They may believe that their disease is a punishment for wrongdoing, or that they have caused their parents to be upset. They may fear abandonment or pain and they may worry about what will become of the family pet. Leaving or creating a legacy is a concern of many children who fear being forgotten.

Good communication is best achieved in the context of an established and trusting relationship. Creating such an environment requires a significant investment of time and energy. Children respond best to people who show an interest in their hobbies, interests and feelings. Sitting with a child and asking about their play and their world is an effective way of understanding them and laying the groundwork for future discussions.

Listening is the most critical element. What does the child already understand of his or her situation? What are their worries? What is it they want to know? Rather than burdening the child with information they do not need or want, these questions can be used to guide a discussion about their key concerns. It may take time for a child to engage in such a discussion and some will never be able to address difficult issues directly. Stories, drawings and play can all facilitate communication in this setting by allowing the child to speak about issues of illness and death as they relate to someone else (e.g. a doll).

### Helping the parents to help the child

Parents are best placed to talk with their child about issues related to death and dying, but understandably many feel anxious about this. Where parents feel strongly that their child should not be informed about the nature of the illness but the child is showing signs of needing to know more, it may be helpful to take the following steps.

▶ Explore with the parents their concerns. What do they think will happen if they speak with the child?
▶ Provide information so that the parents can make an informed decision. Parents need to know that:
  — children generally know a great deal about the condition but may have misconceptions and may be protecting their parents
  — if they are unable to share their worries, children are likely to feel isolated and anxious
  — children are often worried about things about which parents can provide reassurance (e.g. that they will be in pain or be alone)
  — parents who have talked with their children openly rarely regret it; parents who do not, often regret it.[51]
▶ Provide the parents with advice on how to initiate a conversation. It may be helpful to do this through role play.
▶ Offer to be with the parents to help and support them.
▶ If parents still feel unable to speak with the child, suggest alternatives. For example, could a family friend, relative or staff member take on this role? Could another person act as an intermediary between the child and the parents?

Open communication is an ideal – it is not an absolute requirement. For some families who are used to a more closed communication style, enforcing an alternative may be harmful. It is also critical to respect cultural differences.

### Decision-making

Children are largely dependent on others to make sound decisions on their behalf. In the palliative care setting these decisions determine not only whether the child lives or dies but whether or not they are able to access the physical, emotional and spiritual support they need. In general, this responsibility falls to parents, but their decisions are based on the information and advice given to them by the health professionals involved. There are many stakeholders, and each brings a range of factors to the decision-making process.

In the majority of cases there is agreement between all parties on the best way forward. On occasions, however, the interests of the parents and the interests of the child diverge. Distressed parents, desperate for their child to survive, may be unable to acknowledge the suffering of the child and may be unwilling to forgo life-sustaining interventions that afford only a net burden to the child. Less frequently, parents may request that an intervention which is clearly in the child's interest be withheld or withdrawn. In these circumstances, the treating team must advocate very strongly for the child.

### Example

The palliative care team provide advice on symptom management and help with bathing. They are also able to offer music therapy, which Carl clearly enjoys. They understand that the parents cannot agree about Carl's treatment and take the view that with time and ongoing discussion this is likely to resolve. Carl's father will not discuss the matter with any of the team members.

One evening Carl becomes ill very suddenly with a respiratory infection. He is admitted to hospital but the staff there are of the firm view that Carl is dying and would suffer if he were subjected to ventilation. They inform the family that they will treat Carl's infection very actively with antibiotics and oxygen but they will also administer morphine to ease his feelings of dyspnea. Carl's father is very distressed and cries, saying he could never make a decision to end Carl's life. The staff reassure him that sometimes being a good parent means knowing what not to do. The family gathers and there is a long vigil by Carl's bedside. The following morning he shows signs of improvement. He survives this episode and dies six months later of a respiratory infection.

Even very young children can be involved in decision-making to the extent that their developmental level and cognitive capacity allow. For children with chronic illness, this has the added benefit of helping them develop a capacity for decision-making that will be useful later on. Four levels of involvement in decision-making have been described:[52]
1. being informed
2. being consulted
3. having views taken into account in decision-making
4. being respected as the main decision-maker.

Where the child's perspectives on their illness and treatment are solicited, they often provide insights that guide parents in their decision-making. Health professionals can facilitate this process by creating an environment where children feel supported to reveal their thoughts and worries. Children may be able to make some decisions about their medical care (e.g. venepuncture sites) even when major decisions are made by others. Empowering children in this way gives them a sense of control that has a positive impact on their experience of care.

## How siblings react to an ill child

The impact of fatal illness on siblings is profound. Many of their needs for information and support parallel those of the sick child, and they too are dependent on the adults in their lives for support and guidance. Indeed, a heightened need for physical and emotional closeness and the comfort of routine comes at a time when parents are least able to provide such things.

The siblings of children with life-threatening conditions universally experience distress, but few share these feelings with others.[53] They often sense that their parents are already burdened enough and may try to protect them from additional worry. This may account for the fact that parents frequently underestimate the impact on siblings.[53] There may also be an incorrect assumption that a child who does not ask questions does not want information. Siblings who are unable to share their concerns may express grief and distress indirectly through developmental regression, academic failure and social withdrawal.

### Example

Six weeks after Carl's death, his sister Amelia is caught stealing money from another child's bag at school. She tells a counselor at the school that no-one has asked her how she feels about her brother's death. There is a family meeting at which her mother expresses regret, saying that she was so caught up in all of the tasks required of her that she was unable to attend to her daughter's needs. Carl's sister expresses anger that she was not included in his care and was not informed of his prognosis. Her mother cries and says she was just trying to protect her.

Siblings may form incorrect assumptions about the nature of the disease and its cause, causing them to fear for their own health and the health of their parents. Young children may even believe that they caused the illness through some act or omission. Others may feel jealous of the attention received by the sick child and then guilt for having such feelings.

There are even situations where, due to the inherited nature of a condition, multiple children in the same family are affected by a particular condition. In such circumstances, a younger less-affected sibling may witness, over time, the demise of their older brother or sister.

## Section 3: Adults as carers

*Geoffrey Mitchell and Judith Murray*

The presence of a life-limiting illness changes the relationship between people. There is a transition that takes place from an equal relationship between adults to one characterized by dependence of one on another. Seamark and Seamark in Chapter 4 illustrate what the person with the illness experiences as a result of the transition. Here we will observe what happens to the other person. The relationship may be that of spouse or partner, or child and parent where the parent is ill. Less commonly it can be the other way around, where a younger adult may contract a fatal condition and the parents revert to a caring role.

Waldrop and colleagues have studied this group of people and have devised a model that explains the transitions that take place. They based their study on two theoretical perspectives.[54] The first is the concept of a *caregiving career*, described by Pearlin.[55] This theory describes three stages in the career.

1. *Role acquisition* – the carer moves towards a process of care, frequently not being really aware they are assuming the caring role until they are firmly entrenched in it.
2. *Role enactment* – the person goes through the process of caring for their ill loved one.
3. *Role disengagement* – the caregiver relinquishes the role when the ill person dies. It involves a phase of bereavement and adjustment, as outlined above.

The transitions from one phase of the career to the next can prove troublesome in their own right.

Pearlin also proposes a stress process model. This model describes the experiences of the patient as *primary stressors* and *secondary stressors*. Primary stressors are those things that impact on the caregiver directly and are directly attributable to the process of care, while secondary stressors are the impacts of caregiving on other parts of the caregiver's life, including economic strains, lifestyle interference and impacts on other family members. The effects of these stressors are influenced by the social, financial and internal personality resources at the individual's disposal.[56] The concept of primary and secondary stressors is discussed in more detail below.

### Primary stressors

Waldrop has identified a series of experiences common to many carers of adult patients, which equate to Pearlin's primary stressors. They are: comprehending the terminal state of the patient, near-acute care, executive functioning, and final decision-making.

### *Comprehension of the patient's terminal state*

After acquiring the caregiver role, there comes a time when the caregiver develops an increasing comprehension that this illness is likely to lead to imminent death. The caregiver develops this understanding through observation, and through receiving and assimilating information from a range of sources.

This realization may come through information imparted by the practitioner. Some practitioners are quite open about prognosis. Others are far less comfortable revealing this news, and the information comes subtly if at all. The demeanor of the doctor caring for the patient, or words used that aren't quite as positive as previously, may be the only clues. There may be a single precipitous event, where the terminal nature of the illness is clearly spelt out in an investigation finding or a clearly defined medical event like a pathological fracture. This is clearly a shocking realization for the caregiver.

A steady physical decline in the individual is a clear sign of the irreversibility of the process. The patient may require steadily increasing doses or numbers of medications. There may be an increasing number of physical insults (e.g. patients requiring increasingly frequent blood transfusions or peritoneal taps to remove ascitic fluid). Sometimes it is an action or a statement of the patient themselves that conveys to the caregiver that the patient is aware of impending death. The realization may also come as the caregiver notes personality and behavioural changes associated with the patient disengaging from his or her social world.

Once the carer realizes the condition is terminal, there are consequences for other parts of the relationship.

### Near acute care

The level of care the patient requires increases substantially as the illness progresses. As death approaches, more symptoms develop and more quickly, creating rapidly fluctuating clinical situations and complex care needs. The carer is required to do more, both in terms of physical care and managing more complex treatment regimes. There may be increasing visits to (or from) doctors and other professionals. Many patients suffer sleep reversal, where they doze during the day and are awake at night. Carers whose circadian rhythm is intact find themselves up day and night. This can lead to exhaustion and may be the precipitant for inpatient admission.

### Executive functioning

As the patient moves closer to death, the carer of necessity assumes more responsibility for decision-making. The carer finds him-or herself having to make the decisions while at the same time trying to allow the patient the dignity of maintaining his or her traditional role in the decision-making process. However, the role delineation found in couples breaks down as the ill person becomes less capable or less interested in making decisions, or in sharing in joint decisions. The carer picks up more and more responsibility as a result.

*Final decision-making*

This responsibility also extends to making health-related decisions, and decisions relating to the final days of the patient's life. Issues such as when or if to hospitalize, when to withdraw from chemotherapy and calling in extra help are made worse by the realization that each extra decision is a sign that death is one step closer. While some patients plan ahead, often funeral arrangements such as who conducts the service and the details of the service may have to be made by the carer.

## Secondary stressors

Pearlin's secondary stressors equate to one element of the distal context in the patient-centered model. These are stressors created by the illness but external to the carer themselves. They comprise issues such as family tensions, role conflicts, financial strains and work pressures.

Families whose relationships were strained before a major illness may find the relationships brought closer together. However, the tensions can also be exacerbated. In particular, the roles people play within the family can be modified by illness, creating tension.[57] The caregiver role, for example, may be forced on people who may not want it. Caregiving for most is an expected role, and most people accept it without really understanding what will be involved.[58] Finally, tensions between the caregiver role and roles outside the family, like work roles, may lead to significant stress. Coristine[59] found that the caregivers of advanced breast cancer patients assumed the caregiving role until it encroached unacceptably on work time. Alternative arrangements have to be made at that point.

## Example

Wilhelm is a 54-year-old car salesman. His wife, Dorothy, has had breast cancer for two years, which was found to have disseminated six months ago. She has undertaken chemotherapy in an attempt to arrest the disease. However, this has proved fruitless, and the effort of the 60-kilometer round trip for therapy has left her exhausted. Wilhelm has used up all his holiday time helping her on these weekly trips.

She is starting to require full-time care at home. There are children – an older daughter, Fay, who is married with two young children and one on the way, and two boys who are both working full time. All help when they can. Wilhelm can't afford to take any more time off work. He fears that if he takes leave without pay he will lose his job. Times are tough and there is a downturn in the car industry.

Wilhelm's problem was overcome with the help of a volunteer hospice service.

They cared for Dorothy at home during working hours for the final few weeks of her life, and Wilhelm was able to keep his job.

Financial strains are considerable with chronic illness.[60] While insurance schemes and government support will cover the majority of expenses, they often don't account for all the costs. In addition, caring for an ill relative imposes an opportunity cost: if a person is caring they may not be earning. Employment may have to be sacrificed if the carer's employer is unable or unwilling to grant the required time off.

## Modulating influences
### Spirituality, religious faith and faith communities
Spirituality has been defined as:

> . . . a person's unique search . . . for what is sacred in life, answers to life's ultimate questions (such as the meaning, purpose, and direction in life), as well as a feeling of connectedness to others and the environment.[61]

Spirituality is the means by which humans satisfy the need to transcend or rise above the everyday material or sensory experience. It also relates to a person's relationship to God or some higher universal power, force or energy. It is the means by which a person searches for greater meaning, purpose and direction in living, and can also be the framework through which a person seeks non-physical kinds of intervention to provide healing. It provides a framework within which such questions can be answered, and hope derived.[62]

For some, that framework will be related to faith in a higher being. For others, it is confidence in elements of the here and now. Spirituality may promote a sense of calm and security, which can have tangible benefits such as reducing anxiety and depression, speeding recovery from illness, reducing pain, and improving adjustment to disability, to name a few.[63]

Spirituality and religion are frequently thought of as synonyms. They are not. In contrast to spirituality, religion has been defined as:

> . . . an organized system of beliefs, practices, rituals, and symbols designed to facilitate a relationship to and understanding of a deity (or deities) as well as to promote understanding and harmony of a person's relationship to oneself and others in living together in community. Religion as a social institution involves many practices and procedures that have both positive and negative effects.[61]

Religion can be an organizing element, an identifiable marker of many cultures, yet the majority of the population may not be spiritual. The presence of a deity and a relationship with an organized religious community can be particularly significant. For example, in the USA, a study of women with gynecological cancers sought to understand their ways of coping with their illness. Eighty-five percent of women identified with a religious faith, religion was taken seriously by 76%, 49% felt their faith had increased as a result of their illness (none said it had decreased), and 93% said their religious experiences helped sustain their hopes.[64] Similar findings have been reported for melanoma suffers in the USA[65] and Israel.[66]

It is clear that religiosity and spirituality exist as separate, relatively independent dimensions. Thus, people can be both religious and spiritual to different degrees. Those who are both very religious and very spiritual use their spirituality to give meaning and comfort to their situations, expressed in the terms of their particular religious creed. People can also be spiritual yet not religious, ascribing meaning and comfort in terms not specific to a particular religion. People can be religious yet not very spiritual – 'going through the motions' of a religious tradition without necessarily being comforted by it. Others, of course, will not have any interest in the spiritual dimension, and will not subscribe to any religious paradigm.

The patient's and carer's religious and faith practice can play a major part in the experience of illness. In many cases this impact is very positive.[67,68] For example, certainty in an afterlife or a relationship with God can be very reassuring for some. Patients and carers can receive much comfort and support from a minister, priest or other religious representative. Active membership in a faith community can be of immense psychological and practical support.

Conversely, a person's faith may act as a hindrance.[69–72] If the patient or carer perceives the illness to be a consequence of past actions, then there may be little comfort derived from a creed that sees the illness as justified. The person must grit their teeth and bear the punishment. If the illness is seen as punishment, then there may be a reluctance to moderate the symptoms present, symptoms the patient sees as just punishment.

Some patients believe that they will receive divine healing. If the healing doesn't eventuate, they or their fellow believers may attribute the non-healing to a lack of faith. For a person who has a longstanding faith this is a bitter pill to take. As a corollary, some people suffer far more than is necessary through refusal to accept normal treatment. Acceptance of such treatment is perceived by them as denial that God will heal. This can be a source of severe frustration, particularly if this decision is made on behalf of, and not by, the patient.

### Example

Tommy is a 12-year-old boy with an incurable Wilm's tumor. The tumor is increasing in size and causing significant pain. Tommy can hardly move. Dr Tony is calling in regularly to monitor the situation. He dearly wants to start giving him an opioid. However, Tommy's father repeatedly refuses the offer. The family's faith is centered around a belief in the healing power of God, and to resort to treatments like that would be to deny that God will heal his son. All Dr Tony (a committed Christian himself) can do is to suggest that healing comes in many forms, including what a doctor can offer. It is all to no avail, and distressing in the extreme to watch Tommy suffering needlessly.

Practitioners carrying out their daily duties will constantly be confronted with a diverse range of personal perceptions of spirituality, many of which will be very different from their own. They will need to work out how to determine the level of importance the patient and carer attach to spiritual issues, and how these are expressed. They will then have to devise strategies to facilitate the benefits that person's approach can bring to the management of palliative care problems.

### Social and family support

Having a caregiver at home is important. Dying people who live alone are more likely to die in an institution, have higher levels of distress and have less access to specialist palliative care services, and are less likely to die at home than those with a primary caregiver at home.[73]

Social support from other sources at first glance appears vital to the wellbeing of carers and the chance of a suitable outcome for the patient. The help of close family members seems to be invaluable: this help may be the difference between the caregiver managing the situation, or not. As in the case of Wilhelm and Dorothy, external help enabled Wilhelm to keep his job and for Dorothy to be cared for at home. However, having social support is not an important predictor of the ability of the caregiver to cope with the demands of palliative care patients. Heightened anxiety, in conjunction with a poor perceived level of competence at the outset of a referral to a palliative care service, are the best predictors of poor psychosocial functioning in the immediate caregiver.[74] These people will need greater professional support to get through.

## References

1 Miller ED, Omarzu J. New directions in loss research. In: Harvey JH, editor. *Perspectives on Loss: a sourcebook.* Philadelphia: Brunner/Mazel; 1998.
2 MacIntosh D. Suffering and the 'acceptability gap': a clinically useful definition of suffering. Paper presented at the 5th Australian Palliative Care Conference, Brisbane, Australia; 1999.
3 Hegarty M. The dynamic of hope: hoping in the face of death. *Prog Palliat Care.* 2001; 9: 42–6.
4 Hogg KE, Goldstein LH, Leigh PN. The psychological impact of motor neurone disease. *Psychol Med.* 1994; 24(3): 625–32.

5 Olshansky S. Chronic sorrow: a response to having a mentally defective child. *Soc Casework*. 1962; **43**: 190–3.

6 Teel L. Chronic sorrow: analysis of the concept. *J Adv Nurs*. 1991; **16**(11): 1311–19.

7 Lindgren CL, Burke ML, Hainsworth MA, *et al*. Chronic sorrow: a lifespan concept. *Sch Inq Nurs Pract*. 1992; **6**(1): 27–42.

8 McWhinney I. Chapter 6: Illness, suffering and healing. In: McWhinney IR. *A Textbook of Family Medicine*. New York: Oxford University Press; 1989.

9 Burke ML. Chronic sorrow in mothers of school age children with a myelomeningocele disability. *Dissertat Abs Int*. 1989; **50**: 233–48.

10 Garber J, Miller SM, Abramson LY. On the distinction between anxiety and depression: perceived control, certainty and the probability of goal attainment. In: Garber JS, Seligman MEP, editors. *Human Helplessness: theory and applications*. New York: Academic Press; 1980.

11 Abramson L, Metalsky G, Alloy L. Hopelessness depression: a theory-based subtype of depression. *Psychol Rev*. 1989; **96**(2): 358–72.

12 Brown GW, Harris TO, Hepworth C. Loss, humiliation, and entrapment among women developing depression. In: Jenkins JM, Oatley K, Stein NL, editors. *Human Emotions: a reader*. Massachusetts: Blackwell Publishers Inc.; 1995.

13 Creed F, Ash G. Depression in rheumatoid arthritis: aetiology and treatment. *Int Rev Psychiat*. 1992; **4**: 23–34.

14 Lloyd-Williams M. Why are we reluctant to diagnose depression in palliative care patients? *Prog Palliat Care*. 2001; **9**(3): 85–6.

15 Paolucci S, Antonucci G, Grasso MG, *et al*. Post-stroke depression, antidepressant treatment and rehabilitation results. *Cerebrovasc Dis*. 2001; **12**: 264–71.

16 Kimmel PL. Depression in patients with chronic renal disease: what we know and what we need to know. *J Psychosom Res*. 2002; **53**: 951–6.

17 Humphrey GM, Zimpfer DG. *Counselling for Grief and Bereavement*. London: Sage; 1996.

18 Mitchell G. Killing George with kindness: is there such a thing as too much palliative care? *Aust Family Physician*. 2005; **34**: 290–1.

19 Mitchell K, Owens G. End of life decision-making by New Zealand general practitioners: a national survey. *NZ Med J*. 2004; **117**(1196): U934.

20 Marquet R, Bartelds A, Visser G, *et al*. Twenty-five years of requests for euthanasia and physician assisted suicide in Dutch general practice: trend analysis. *BMJ* 2003; **327**: 201–2.

21 Erikson E. *Childhood and Society*. New York: Norton; 1950.

22 Haight BK. Reminiscing: the state of the art as a basis for practice. *Int J Aging Hum Devt*. 1991; **33**(1): 1–32.

23 Hatchett L, Friend R, Symister P, *et al*. Interpersonal expectations, social support, and adjustment to chronic illness. *J Personality and Soc Psychol*. 1997; **73**(3): 560–73.

24 Ingram RE, Hamilton NA. Evaluating precision in the social psychological assessment of depression: methodological considerations, issues, and recommendations. *J Soc Clin Psychol*. 1999; **18**(2): 160–80.

25 Symister P, Friend R. The influence of social support and problematic support on optimism and depression in chronic illness: a prospective study evaluating self-esteem as a mediator. *Health Psychol*. 2003; **22**(2): 123–9.

26 Bass DM, Bowman K. The transition from caregiving to bereavement: the relationship of care-related strain and adjustment to death. *Gerontologist*. 1990; **30**(1): 35–42.

27 Bass DM, Bowman K, Noelker LS. The influence of caregiving and bereavement support on adjusting to an older relative's death. *Gerontologist.* 1991; **31**(1): 32–42.

28 Rando T. An investigation of grief and adaptation in parents whose children have died from cancer. *J Ped Psychol.* 1983; **8**: 3–19.

29 Middleton W, Raphael B, Burnett P, *et al.* A longitudinal study comparing bereavement phenomena in recently bereaved spouses, adult children and parents. *Aust NZ J Psychiat.* 1998; **32**: 235–41.

30 Hazzard A, Weston J, Gutterres C. After a child's death: factors related to parental bereavement. *J Dev Behav Pediatr.* 1992; **13**: 24–30.

31 Li J, Precht D, Mortensen P. Mortality in parents after death of a child in Denmark: nationwide follow-up study. *Lancet* 2003; **361**: 363–7.

32 Spinetta J, Murphy J, Vik P, *et al.* Long-term adjustment in families of children with cancer. *J Psychosocial Onc.* 1988; **6**: 179–91.

33 Davies B, Deveau E, de Veber B, *et al.* Experiences of mothers in five countries whose child died of cancer. *Cancer Nurs.* 1998; **21**: 301–11.

34 Mastroyannopoulou KSP, Lewis M, Lenton S. The impact of childhood non-malignant life-threatening illness on parents: gender differences and predictors of parental adjustment. *J Psychol Psychiatr.* 1997; **38**: 823–9.

35 Sloper P. Needs and responses of parents following the diagnosis of childhood cancer. *Child Care Health Dev.* 1996; **22**: 187–202.

36 Dockerty J, Skegg D, Williams S. Economic effects of childhood cancer on families. *J Paed Child Health.* 2003; **39**: 254–8.

37 Dangel T, Fowler-Kerry S, Karwacki M, *et al.* An evaluation of a home palliative care programme for children. *J Ambulat Child Health.* 2000; **2000**: 101–16.

38 Lenton S, Stallard P, Mastroyannopoulou K. Prevalence and morbidity associated with non-malignant, life-threatening conditions in childhood. *Child Care Health Dev.* 2001; **27**: 389–98.

39 Sirkia K, Saarinen U, Ahlgren B, *et al.* Terminal care of the child with cancer at home. *Acta Pediatr.* 1997; **100**: 1125–30.

40 Lauer M, Mulhern R, Wallskog J, *et al.* A comparison study of parental adaptation following a child's death at home or in hospital. *Pediatrics.* 1983; **71**: 107–12.

41 Lauer M, Camitta B. Home care for dying children: a nursing model. *J Pediatrics.* 1980; **97**: 1032–5.

42 Collins J, Stevens M, Cousens P. Home care for the dying child. *Aust Family Physician.* 1998; **27**: 610–14.

43 Wray D, Wray S. Andrew: a journey – a parent's perspective. *Child Care Health Dev.* 2004; **30**: 201–2.

44 Davies B, Gudmundsdottir M, Worden W, *et al.* 'Living in the dragon's shadow': fathers' experiences of a child's life-limiting illness. *Death Stud.* 2004; **28**: 111–35.

45 Steele R. Trajectory of certain death at an unknown time: children with neurodegenerative life-threatening illnesses. *Can J Nurs Res.* 2000; **32**: 49–67.

46 Wheeler I. Parental bereavement: the crisis of meaning. *Death Stud.* 2001; **25**: 51–66.

47 Kellehear A. Grief and loss: past, present and future. *Med J Aust.* 2002; **177**: 176–7.

48 Beale E, Baile W, Aaron J. Silence is not golden: communicating with children dying from cancer. *J Clin Oncol.* 2005; **23**: 3629–31.

49 Waechter E. Children's awareness of fatal illness. *Am J Nursing.* 1971; **71**: 1168–72.

50 Adams-Greenly M. Helping children communicate about serious illness and death. *J Psychosocial Onc.* 1984; **2**: 61–72.

51 Kreicbergs U, Valdimarsdottir U, Onelov E, *et al.* Talking about death with children who have severe malignant disease. *N Engl J Med.* 2004; **351**: 1175–86.

52 Royal College of Paediatrics and Child Health. *Withholding and Withdrawing Life Sustaining Treatment in Children: a framework for practice.* 2nd edition. London: RCPCH; London 2004.

53 Stallard P, Mastroyannopoulou K, Lewis M, *et al.* The siblings of children with life-threatening conditions. *Child Psychol Psychiatr Rev.* 1997; **2**: 823–9.

54 Waldrop DP, Kramer BJ, Skretny JA, *et al.* Final transitions: family caregiving at the end of life. *J Palliat Med.* 2005; **8**: 623–38.

55 Pearlin LI. The careers of caregivers. *Gerontologist.* 1992; **32**: 647.

56 Pearlin LI, Aneshensel CS. Caregiving: the unexpected career. *Soc Justice Res.* 1994; **7**: 373–90.

57 Manne SL, Alfieri T, Taylor KL, *et al.* Spousal negative responses to cancer patients: the role of social restriction, spouse mood, and relationship satisfaction. *J Consult Clin Psychol.* 1999; **67**: 352–61.

58 Berg-Weger M. Role induction and caregiver strain: a structural equation approach. *J Soc Service Res.* 1995; **21**: 33–53.

59 Coristine M, Crooks D, Grunfeld E, *et al.* Stonebridge C., Christie A. Caregiving for women with advanced breast cancer. *Psychooncology* 2003; 12: 709–19.

60 Barg FK, Pasacreta JV, Nuamah IF, *et al.* A description of a psychoeducational intervention for family caregivers of cancer patients. *J Family Nurs.* 1998; **4**: 394–413.

61 Larson D, Sawyers J, McCullough M. *Scientific Research on Spirituality and Health: a consensus report.* Rockville, MD: National Institute for Healthcare Research; 1997.

62 Aldridge D. Spirituality, healing and medicine. *Br J General Pract.* 1993; **41**: 425–7.

63 Post S, Puchalski C, Larson D. Physicians and patient spirituality: professional boundaries, competency and ethics. *Ann Int Med.* 2000; **132**: 578–83.

64 Roberts JA, Brown D, Elkins T, *et al.* Factors influencing views of patients with gynecologic cancer about end-of-life decisions. *Am J Obstet Gynecol.* 1997; **176**: 166–72.

65 Holland JC, Passik S, Kash KM, *et al.* The role of religious and spiritual beliefs in coping with malignant melanoma. *Psychooncology* 1999; **8**: 14–26.

66 Balder L, Russack SM, Perry S, *et al.* The role of spiritual and religious beliefs in coping with malignant melanoma: an Israeli sample. *Psychooncology* 1999; **8**: 27–35.

67 George LK, Larson DB, Koenig HG, *et al.* Spirituality and health: what we know, what we need to know. *J Soc Clin Psychol.* 2000; **19**(1): 102–16.

68 Mytko JJ, Knight SJ. Body, mind and spirit: towards the integration of religiosity and spirituality in cancer quality of life research. *Psychooncology* 1999; **8**: 439–50.

69 Koenig HG. *Is Religion Good for Your Health?: the effects of religion on physical and mental health.* New York: Haworth Pastoral Press; 1997.

70 Pargament KI, Zinnbauer BJ, Scott AB, *et al.* Red flags and religious coping: identifying some religious warning signs among people in crisis. *J Clin Psychol.* 1998; **59**: 1335–48.

71 Berecz JM. All that glitters is not gold: bad forgiveness in counseling and preaching. *Pastoral Psychol.* 2001; **49**: 253–75.

72 Jenkins RA, Pargament KI. Religion and spirituality as resources for coping with cancer: psychosocial resource variables in cancer studies. In: Curbow B, Somerfield MR, editors. *Concept Measure Issues.* 1995; 13: 51–74.

73 Aoun S, Kristjanson LJ, Currow D, *et al*. Terminally ill people living alone without a caregiver: an Australian national scoping study of palliative care needs. *Palliat Med.* 2007; **21**: 29–34.

74 Hudson PL, Hayman-White K, Aranda S, *et al*. Predicting family caregiver psychosocial functioning in palliative care. *J Palliat Care.* 2006; **22**: 133–40.

# CHAPTER 6

# Symptom management in palliative care

*PATSY YATES, JANET HARDY*

## Introduction

Palliative care is a specialized area of healthcare that has emerged to respond to the experiences and needs of people with life-limiting illness. Palliative care has been defined by the World Health Organization (WHO) as:

> . . . an approach that improves the quality of life of patients and their families facing problems associated with life-threatening illness, through the prevention of suffering by means of early identification and impeccable assessment and treatment of pain and other problems, physical, psychological and spiritual. (*World Health Organization (WHO) definition of palliative care, 2004*)*

Consistent with this definition, a number of key principles can be identified to underpin a person-centered approach to clinical management in palliative care. These principles include:

▶ the palliative approach is identified as being relevant early in the course of an illness, not just as end-of-life care
▶ palliative care promotes holistic care to ensure physical, psychological, social and spiritual well-being
▶ the family and significant others are included in the care process

---

* www.who.int/cancer.palliative/definition/en. Accessed October 2004.

) there is an emphasis on impeccable assessment, early identification of problems and implementation of appropriate treatments

) disease-modifying treatments, such as chemotherapy and radiotherapy, may have a role

) palliative care can be provided in any setting

) there is an emphasis on a team approach to care.

In this chapter, Yates and Hardy introduce Adrian, a man dying of disseminated melanoma, and show how these principles can be applied to managing some of the more common clinical problems that arise in palliative care. The chapter focuses on managing common symptoms including pain, dyspnea, nausea, fatigue and anorexia. Management issues associated with other important and related care needs, such as psychological distress and spiritual concerns, are addressed elsewhere in this book.

For clarity, each of the symptoms addressed in this chapter is described separately. As seen in Adrian's case, however, patients are more likely to present with several concurrent symptoms. The complex interrelationships between these various symptoms should be considered when identifying an appropriate management plan.

## Adrian

Adrian is a 30-year-old, previously well male who works for a mortgage company. He is married to Christie and they have two small children, aged three and six. Three years previously, a level 3 melanoma was excised from his back. Following the initial incision of the mole by his GP, he underwent a wider excision by a surgeon in the private sector. Histology of the wider resection was clear and he has had no regular follow-up since.

In March he presented to his GP with back pain, initially thought to have resulted from a rugby injury. Plain X-rays were unremarkable and he was reassured. The back pain continued, however, and he was having increasing periods of sick leave from work. A diagnosis of 'stress' secondary to work-related pressures was made. When a mass developed in his left axilla in May, he was referred for an urgent oncology opinion. A fine-needle aspirate of the axillary node was positive for carcinoma, consistent with metastatic melanoma. A bone scan showed multiple areas of increased uptake consistent with wide-spread bone metastases. A staging CT scan also revealed multiple small lung metastases.

He began chemotherapy (dacarbazine) and radiotherapy to the lower lumbar spine. A repeat CT scan following two courses of chemotherapy revealed no response, with progression of his lung and liver disease and the development of a pleural effusion. On review he complained of increasing pain in the abdomen and upper back, with pain radiating around the chest wall, as well as dyspnea, nausea and a lack of appetite. His GP prescribed slow release tramadol for pain and metoclopramide 10mg tds for nausea. Routine blood tests revealed worsening liver function tests and hypercalcemia. The chemotherapy was discontinued, and he was referred to palliative care.

## Understanding the person's experience of symptoms

Symptoms can be defined as 'subjective experience[s] reflecting changes in the bio-psychosocial functioning, sensations, or cognition of an individual'.[1] Such definitions highlight that symptoms are subjective and multidimensional. The nature of many life-limiting conditions also means that symptoms don't always follow a predictable pattern. Moreover, the management of clinical problems and symptoms associated with life-limiting illnesses may be different, depending on whether the person presents with the problem early in the course of their illness or at a later stage. Understanding how to manage these complex palliative problems from a person-centered perspective requires an appreciation of the unique features of an individual's symptom experience.

Symptoms comprise an individual's perception (whether a person notices a change in the way he or she usually feels), evaluation (one's judgement about the severity, cause, treatability and effect of symptoms on their lives), as well as responses to the symptom (the physical, psychological, sociocultural and behavioural pain components).[1] These perceptions, evaluations and responses can be influenced by a range of personal, environmental and health- or illness-related factors. For example, experiences of dyspnea may vary according to the underlying pathology and etiology of the symptom,[2] and a person's evaluation of the meaning of their fatigue may depend on their views about whether the fatigue is related to the progression of their disease or some other non-disease-related factor.[3] Similarly, how a person responds to their pain can be influenced by a range of sociocultural beliefs and expectations.[4]

Because of the complex nature of symptoms, their subjectivity and the enormous variability in individual perceptions, evaluations and responses, the management of these problems typically requires a multifaceted and individ-ualized response. Some key principles for symptom management that will be explored in the remainder of this chapter include that effective management of symptoms requires:

- an integrated approach, which may include interventions aimed at one or more of the components of the symptom (e.g. the use of pharmacological as well as non-pharmacological measures)
- a targeted approach to ensure it is directed at specific causal mechanisms and/ or the social, psychological or spiritual factors contributing to the problem

◗ a tailored approach to ensure it is suitable to the person's circumstances, beliefs, goals and preferences.[5]

## Pain

A detailed pain history and examination in Adrian's case reveals several sites and types of pain, as is typical of most patients with advanced cancer.[6] The pain that is worrying Adrian and his wife, Christie, most is the pain in his upper back, especially because it is so similar to the pain that led to the diagnosis of his metastatic disease. His description is of pain, sited over the upper thoracic vertebrae, with focal tenderness. This is typical of mechanical nociceptive pain secondary to bone metastases in the spine following destruction of bone by tumour. The pain is exacerbated by movement or coughing, and can thus be described as incident pain. His sleep has been disturbed because it is painful to lie on his back. Adrian and Christie have been forced to sleep in different rooms because Adrian's nights have been so disturbed.

He also describes an unpleasant aching pain radiating around the left chest wall from the back at nipple level, with skin hyper-sensitivity. This is characteristic of neuropathic pain resulting from nerve damage, infiltration or compression. This type of pain is often described as an unpleasant aching sensation that can occasionally be shooting or lancinating and is often associated with weakness and/or sensory changes (either hyperesthesia or numbness). This history is very suggestive of nerve root involvement by tumour infiltrating the upper thoracic vertebrae or compressing the nerve root.

Adrian points to a third site of pain in the upper abdomen. Liver metastases often present as a feeling of fullness or discomfort in the right upper quadrant of the abdomen. A bleed into a liver metastasis with involvement of the liver capsule can cause severe upper quadrant pain that generally resolves with time.

As well as the multi-site physical pain from advanced cancer, this young man is also likely to be experiencing 'spiritual' pain as a consequence of his fear, anger, and uncertainty regarding the future. He has a wife and young children to support and has not been able to work for some months. He finds it difficult to discuss his condition with Christie and 'down plays' many of his symptoms so as not to worry her. He is thus dealing with much of this pain alone. (Issues relating to the non-physical aspects of pain are dealt with in Chapter 3, p. 42)

The goals of pain management are likely to change over time. At first, the goal is to achieve a degree of pain control to allow Adrian to be as mobile and active as possible. With the inevitable progression of his disease and associated reduction in mobility, a more realistic goal at a later stage might be to ensure that he is pain free at rest and that pain is not interfering with his ability to sleep.

This necessitates constant re-evaluation and the ability to change his treatment plan according to his changing condition.

## Pharmacological management

The WHO analgesic ladder provides a relatively simple, easy-to-use analgesic guide that matches drugs to pain severity.[7] Although there has been much recent controversy over its format, and concern that its effectiveness in controlling pain is unproven,[8] the WHO ladder remains the 'gold standard' for the treatment of chronic pain in many countries.

The ladder has three steps for pain of increasing intensity, from mild to severe, and recommends a small number of drugs for use at each step (*see* Figure 6.1). At each step, adjuvant analgesics or co-analgesics can be added. These are drugs whose primary function is not analgesia, but which can confer added analgesic benefit when combined with standard analgesics (e.g. antidepressants when used to treat neuropathic pain (*see* below). The opioid of choice at step 3 of the ladder (severe pain) is morphine. Although there has been a plethora of new opioids

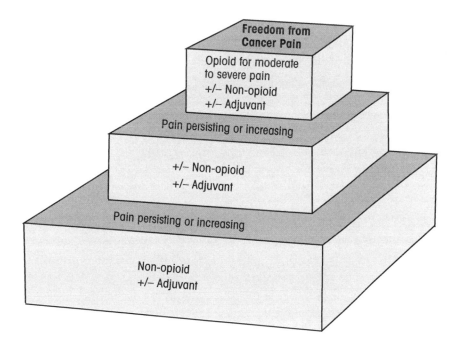

**FIGURE 6.1** The WHO pain relief ladder

Source: World Health Organization. http://www.who.int/cancer/palliative/painladder/en/. Accessed December 22, 2005

and opioid formulations appearing over recent years, there remains no strong evidence of benefit of any one opioid over another.[9] However, some opioids are better suited to individual patients for a variety of reasons, including toxicity, route preference and cost.

Adrian's pain has not been controlled on tramadol (a drug generally classed as a WHO ladder steps 2–3 analgesic), and it would therefore be appropriate to replace this with a 'strong' opioid such as morphine. Routine practice is to start the patient on a normal-release morphine preparation given four-hourly and to convert to an extended-release preparation once the pain control is stable. He is known to be hypercalcemic, however, and is therefore likely to have some impairment of renal function secondary to dehydration. As the major metabolite of morphine is excreted via the kidneys, his dose requirements may be less than anticipated. He would be best suited to an opioid whose excretion is not affected by renal function.

Fentanyl is an ideal drug in this context, but there is no oral preparation of the drug and the transdermal patch preparation is difficult to use for dose titration. Methadone is another opioid not affected by renal function, but this drug has unique dosing properties that make it difficult to use by inexperienced practitioners. Oxycodone, a synthetic opioid, is not metabolized to active metabolites and is probably safer to use in renal impairment than morphine. Titration with immediate-release oxycodone prior to conversion to the delayed-release preparation would be a reasonable option in this case.

When starting any patient on opioids, it is essential to warn them of potential side-effects and to treat these prophylactically.[10] About half of patients starting on opioids will experience nausea and a degree of sedation. This generally resolves within two or three days. Constipation is an almost inevitable consequence of opioid therapy and does not resolve with time. Laxatives (stimulants and softeners rather than bulking agents) should always be prescribed concurrently.

Christie may be concerned that Adrian will become addicted to opioids. It is essential to address these fears and to reassure them both that although Adrian is likely to become physically tolerant to these drugs, addiction implies a psychological need for a drug with associated drug-seeking behaviour that is seen very rarely when opioids are used for the control of pain. Similarly, Adrian may be loath to start strong pain killers in the mistaken belief that there will be nothing left for him when the pain becomes 'really bad'. Although pain in most patients can be controlled on a dose of opioid equivalent to $\leq$ 30 mg morphine four-hourly, it is likely that his opioid requirements will increase with time. This is the result of both the progression of the disease and some degree of tolerance to opioid analgesia. Both must be reassured that there is no upper dose limit for opioids and that they need not fear pain as an inevitable consequence of advanced cancer.

The most appropriate route of opioid delivery is likely to change with time. In the terminal phase, when patients are unable to take medicines by mouth, opioids are usually delivered subcutaneously via a portable syringe driver.

Non-steroidal anti-inflammatories (NSAIDs) have an established role at step 1 of the analgesic ladder and as adjuvant analgesics (*see* below). They are used commonly for bone pain and/or liver pain, although there is no evidence that they are any more effective for this type of pain.[11] It might be of benefit to add an NSAID to Adrian's pain control program, although care should be taken if he has any element of renal impairment. Similarly, it should be discontinued if he is ever started on corticosteroids because this combination increases the risk of gastric irritation 10-fold.

Radiotherapy provides an excellent means of palliating bone pain. Multiple trials have confirmed that single fractions are as efficacious as multiple fractions in palliation, with up to 80% of patients reporting pain relief within two weeks.[12] In this case, the history of mid-back pain suggests further vertebral disease, with encroachment of nerve roots, resulting in the neuropathic pain radiating around the chest wall. Of concern is the possibility of *spinal cord compression*. Ideally, this should be investigated by magnetic resonance imaging (MRI), even in the absence of definitive neurological signs or symptoms, because the consequences of late presentation are devastating. The degree of permanent neurological damage resulting from compression of the spinal cord is directly related to the time at which symptoms first develop and the time to start of treatment.

The appropriateness of radiotherapy will depend on the fitness of the patient at the time. In a young man such as Adrian, where the maintenance of mobility for as long as possible is very important, multiple out-patient visits to the radiotherapy department will be justified. In the later stage of disease, or in patients who are bed-bound, the difficulties inherent in transporting to and from hospital must be weighed against the potential benefits of treatment.

The widespread use of bisphosphonates in recent years for patients with bone metastases has significantly reduced the incidence of pathological fractures and the need for radiotherapy.[13] Responders to bisphosphonates also show an improvement in quality of life.[14] The benefit of bisphosphonates is greater when the duration of treatment is more than six months, so the use of these drugs in an attempt to improve skeletal morbidity must be questioned in patients such as Adrian who are likely to have a short prognosis.

The usual practice when treating neuropathic pain is to determine how much pain relief can be gained from the use of standard analgesics as per the WHO analgesic ladder, but to have a low threshold for co-prescribing a co-analgesic or adjuvant analgesic. These agents have a primary role other than pain relief but can have an additive analgesic effect when used in conjunction with standard analgesics. Those agents for which there is proven evidence of benefit in neuropathic pain include antidepressants[15] and anticonvulsants.[16] These agents have side-effects and contra-indications, however, and the number of patients that must be treated in order for one patient to get a benefit (Number Needed to Treat – NNT) is in the order of three to four.

For a man in his 30s, who is unlikely to have a history of cardiac arrhythmias or urinary retention, a trial of a tricyclic antidepressant such as amitriptyline is a reasonable option if the neuropathic chest wall pain is not relieved by opioids. Some patients find the associated sedation intolerable. It is very important to warn patients of this potential side-effect and to start at a low dose before escalating, although some patients find this beneficial as a sleep aid. They also need to be aware that any beneficial effect may take several weeks to become apparent.

Adrian is now on a number of medications, the doses of which may vary with time and according to response. Many of these drugs will have potential adverse effects and will have been prescribed for indications other than the primary drug indication. It is crucial to spend time with Adrian and Christie to explain exactly when each drug should be taken, what the drug is being prescribed for and what side-effects to expect. The provision of a medicine chart documenting this is often of great benefit to patients and their families. Similarly, a pain chart can be invaluable in plotting and monitoring pain levels on a daily basis.

### Non-pharmacological strategies

Adrian's pain has continued for some time, and may therefore benefit from a range of techniques that involve stimulating cutaneous receptors by pressure (touch or massage) or by temperature (cold or heat) used as adjuncts to pharmacological strategies. While the exact mechanism by which non-pharmacological techniques reduce pain is uncertain, most of these techniques are thought to promote superficial increases in circulation and may counteract the effects of decreased oxygenation and the accumulation of metabolites associated with musculoskeletal pain.[17] They may also help by reducing the anxiety and emotional distress that may exacerbate an individual's pain experience.[18] Contra-indications to using these techniques include bleeding disorders, and other pains characterized by hyperesthesia or hypersensitivity, or broken skin or open wounds. It has also been suggested that deep heat, pressure and vibration should not be used directly on sites with underlying tumour.[17]

Adrian's beliefs about pain and opioids are likely to influence how he responds to pain, including his willingness and ability to report pain and adhere to prescribed therapies. Cognitive–behavioural interventions, including patient education and relaxation techniques, should be considered an integral component of a comprehensive approach to Adrian's pain management. For example, instruction in the effects of prescribed therapies and self-care, and assisting with problem solving, may help overcome concerns Adrian and Christie may have about analgesia as well as provide him with the skills to prevent and manage the side-effects of his medication.[19] Imagery distraction, and relaxation techniques such as imagining images and/or positive emotions, or through the use of audio tapes or music, may also be effective.

A number of these non-pharmacological pain therapies do, however, require active involvement of the patient and their caregivers. Patient motivation is likely to be a critical factor influencing the effectiveness of these approaches, particularly if repeated self-administration is required.[19] As Adrian's illness progresses, his ability and preference for use of such strategies needs to be continually reassessed. Strategies requiring less active involvement, such as music therapy, may be more appropriate at this time. Overall, there is limited evidence on when and how to incorporate non-pharmacological therapies for cancer pain management. Decisions on their use need to be based on clinical judgement, patient preference and assessment of the risk–benefit ratio.[20]

## Nausea

Adrian's reports of nausea require further assessment to understand the potential contributing factors and thereby determine an effective approach to management. Nausea is common in palliative care patients – opioids, liver metastases, hypercalcemia, radiotherapy and constipation are all possible contributors to nausea in this case. In the first instance one would treat any obvious reversible cause. This reflects a targeted, mechanistic approach to the management of nausea, by attempting to identify the most likely cause and treat according to the specific pathophysiology and presumed receptors involved.

However, the exact cause of nausea in advanced cancer is often not clear in these patients and the nausea is often multifactorial.[21] Therefore, an alternative is an empirical approach, whereby an anti-emetic is used irrespective of presumed cause. There is no evidence that one method is better than the other.[21]

### Pharmacological management

The most 'treatable' cause in Adrian's case is likely to be hypercalcemia. Nausea, along with polyuria, polydipsia and drowsiness, is the common presenting symptom of this condition. Rehydration and treatment with bisphosphonates is now the established treatment.[22] Serum calcium levels should return to normal levels within three to five days, as reflected by an improvement in symptoms. The hypercalcemia will recur in three to four weeks, however, unless the underlying malignancy is treated.

The 5HT3 antagonist anti-emetics such as granisetron and ondansetron have a proven role in the control of nausea and vomiting associated with radiotherapy and/or chemotherapy.[23] Ideally, they should be used to cover the period of treatment only, as these drugs will exacerbate constipation, especially in patients on opioids.

The nausea associated with opioids usually resolves within two to three days of starting an opioid or increasing the dose. Many physicians will give an anti-emetic prophylactically when starting opioids. A gastrokinetic such as metoclopramide would be a logical choice, in that the reduction in bowel motility from the use of opioids is thought to contribute to opioid-induced nausea. Others prefer haloperidol, targeting dopamine receptors in the central nervous system. In some cases the nausea does not resolve, in which case one might consider rotating or switching to another opioid in an attempt to improve side-effects.[10] There is no evidence that any one opioid is less likely to cause nausea than another, but some patients will tolerate one opioid better than others.

Constipation is another potentially reversible cause of nausea and is likely to have been exacerbated in this case by the hypercalcemia. Enemata and suppositories might be necessary if the nausea makes it difficult for the patient to tolerate large doses of laxatives by mouth.

There is anecdotal evidence that steroids can improve nausea secondary to liver metastases. Adrian is likely to have been started on steroids because of concern at the possibility of spinal cord compression.

The plan outlined above reflects a targeted, mechanistic approach to the management of nausea, whereby an attempt has been made to identify the most likely cause. However, given that the exact cause of Adrian's nausea may be difficult to determine, and multiple factors could be contributing, an empirical approach may be preferable. In this case, anti-emetics such as metoclopramide or haloperidol would be reasonable options, used irrespective of the presumed cause. Regular assessment of this symptom is crucial. If the nausea is so severe that anti-emetics cannot be taken by mouth, they must be delivered by an alternative route (e.g. sublingually or subcutaneously).

### Non-pharmacological strategies

Environmental stimuli, such as sights, sounds or smells that may initiate Adrian's nausea, should be avoided.[24] For some patients, identifying and avoiding the foods that promote nausea such as fatty, highly salted or spicy foods should also be trialled.[24] Discussions should be held with Christie about ways to plan, prepare and present meals.

There is good evidence that behavioral interventions such as progressive muscle relaxation and guided imagery can control anticipatory nausea and vomiting in patients undergoing cancer chemotherapy. Evidence for the efficacy of behavioral interventions to control post-chemotherapy nausea and vomiting is, however, mixed.[25] Although the extent to which these approaches can be extrapolated to patients with advanced disease is unclear,[26] the positive results noted in patients receiving chemotherapy indicate that these strategies may be useful in the palliative care setting.[24] Adrian's preference and ability to employ such interventions are, however, key considerations as his illness progresses.

## Dyspnea

Dyspnea is a symptom frequently reported by patients with cancer and it can play a central role in their distress. Adrian has a pleural effusion and lung metastases. He is also at high risk of pulmonary emboli (in view of his underlying malignancy) and of chest infections (through chest pain preventing him from expanding his chest fully during inspiration). Adrian's breathlessness is also likely to be causing significant anxiety and distress, and restricting his day-to-day activities.

### Pharmacological management

Drainage of the pleural effusion will give considerable relief, as can anticoagulants and antibiotics when targeting pulmonary emboli or chest infections. The weight of anecdotal evidence supports the use of steroids if the dyspnea is secondary to lymphangitis carcinomatosis or bronchial obstruction. However, if the dyspnea is primarily related to the underlying lung disease, for which there is no further specific anti-cancer therapy, symptom control is more difficult. Standard practice is to prescribe small doses of oral opioids for palliation. The usual practice when palliating breathlessness in a patient such as Adrian, who is already on opioids, is to increase the baseline opioid dose by about 10%.

The benefit of opioids in dyspnea has been confirmed by systematic review of several controlled trials.[27] By contrast, nebulised morphine provides no more relief than nebulised normal saline. Benzodiazepines relieve the often overwhelming anxiety associated with respiratory distress. They can be given sublingually (e.g. lorazepam), orally (diazepam) or subcutaneously in patients unable to take oral medications (midazolam). A common practice is to start with a short-acting benzodiazepine on an 'as required' basis and to convert to a continuous infusion of a parenteral formulation in line with any worsening of the symptom with time and progression of the disease.

### Non-pharmacological strategies

A range of non-drug interventions may also be useful in the management of Adrian's dyspnea. For example, techniques such as 'purse lip' and diaphragmatic breathing can help the patient to slow and control the rate and depth of respiration. This breathing retraining can be utilized by the patient to regain control over breathing and achieve improved alveolar ventilation and oxygenation, increased strength, co-ordination and efficiency of respiratory muscles, and decreased functional residual capacity.[28,29]

A range of other strategies that assist with addressing the anxiety and distress associated with dyspnea, such as relaxation training, distraction and cognitive behavioural techniques, may also be useful.[30,31] For example, discussing Adrian's fears and concerns about dyspnea may provide an opportunity for the health professional to provide emotional support and goal-setting to help in the management of his functional and social activities. It is also likely to improve his quality of life by enabling him to focus on activities he most enjoys.[32] Christie is likely to be distressed by Adrian's dyspnea, and her distress may in turn exacerbate the dyspnea.[33] Involving Christie in supportive activities to help control the breathlessness may help her to cope more effectively.

A recent systematic review has reported highly significant improvements in patients' breathlessness, functional capacity, activity levels and distress levels in a number of studies evaluating non-pharmacological interventions for dyspnea.[34] The overwhelming nature of dyspnea, coupled with the fact that it often worsens as the disease progresses, does, however, mean that ongoing support and encouragement are required. Some patients may simply not have the physical or psychological energy to regain a sense of control over what is happening to them, and feelings of panic associated with breathlessness may be overwhelming.[35]

## Fatigue

The problem of fatigue is often underestimated, despite the fact that it is probably the most common unrelieved symptom of cancer. It interferes significantly with Adrian's ability to interact with his two young children and is a continuing source of concern for Christie. As with other symptoms of advanced disease, the causes are often multifactorial and difficult to determine. Although the multiple etiologies of fatigue highlight the fundamental need to target underlying medical causes (e.g. anemia, hypothyroidism, depression, radiotherapy), there are many less easily treatable factors contributing to the problem that must also be addressed (*see* Chapter 3).

### Pharmacological management

When no obvious reversible cause for fatigue is found, treatment is difficult. Corticosteroids will often improve mood and general well-being, but there is little evidence they improve fatigue. Other pharmacological treatments that have been evaluated include progestogens, anabolic steroids and psychostimulants, but none of these agents have a proven role in this condition. Psychostimulants may have a role when the fatigue is secondary to opioid therapy, especially in young patients (such as in this case).[36]

Depression and associated fatigue are common in cancer patients. The devastating effect of the cancer on Adrian's lifestyle, his inability to carry out daily activities, his fear and relative social isolation will all be contributing to an exogenous depressive state. He has already been started on an antidepressant for treatment of his neuropathic pain, and this may have an added benefit for his mood if the dose is titrated to a sufficiently high level. Depression has been linked to requests for euthanasia,[37] and most clinicians will have a low threshold for instigating antidepressants even in those patients who do not meet all the standard diagnostic criteria.

### Non-pharmacological strategies

Recent systematic reviews report that exercise at low to moderate level customized to the patient's baseline appears to be helpful in improving physical function and resulting in lower fatigue levels for patients during and following cancer treatment.[38] Adrian's breathlessness is likely to restrict activity-based interventions, which may not be feasible in this case and would need to be administered with caution. Few studies have examined when and how to deliver exercise and activity-based interventions to patients with advanced disease.

One recent pilot study of a low- to moderate-intensity seated exercise intervention in patients with advanced disease for whom walking programs may be too intense has shown that the activity-based intervention led to less increase in fatigue and slower decrease in physical quality of life.[39] Principles that may be helpful for Adrian are therefore likely to include minimising unnecessary bed rest, and encouraging continuing previous activity levels for as long as possible.

Attention-restoring activities have been suggested to help to restore the ability to think clearly and enable a person to participate more fully in their care and in life activities.[40] In one study, Cimprich[41] found that women who spent 30 minutes three times weekly using attention-restoring activities showed an increased rate of recovery and of engaging in new activities than the patients in the control group.[41]

As the disease progresses, increasing fatigue and drowsiness may cause added distress to Adrian and Christie. It is important to treat the problems that are disturbing Adrian's sleep (such as his pain) and to ensure that he can optimize his activity and social interactions. For patients whose sleep is affected, strategies to promote a restful sleep may include recommending that they sleep just long enough, wake at the same time each day, avoid stimulants, limit alcohol, and maintain activity levels.

## Anorexia / weight loss

Weight loss can have a profound affect on body image, especially in a young patient such as Adrian, and may cause Christie significant concern. Moreover, once established (over 10% of pre-morbid body weight), cachexia associated with malignancy can be very difficult to reverse.

### Pharmacological strategies

The improvement in appetite and general well-being in trials of corticosteroids was not translated into non-fluid weight gain in many of the earlier trials, although one controlled trial of dexamethasone versus megestrol acetate versus fluoxymesterone in cancer patients with weight loss did show a benefit in favour of both dexamethasone and the progestogen.[42]

Several clinical studies have shown a benefit for both weight gain, appetite and sense of well-being in patients taking progestogens. The effect seems greatest with sustained use of higher-dose therapy. This is not without side-effects (peripheral edema, venous thrombosis, nausea and impotence), however, and is of limited applicability in patients with far advanced disease and a short prognosis. Metoclopramide is recommended in patients with gastric stasis or bowel mobility problems to improve appetite.

### Non-pharmacological strategies

Interventions for the person with cancer who has or is at risk of nutritional problems are directed to increasing caloric and nutritional intake. Interventions to address factors that may be affecting Adrian's intake (such as discomfort and other symptoms) should be implemented. Wherever possible, these interventions should focus on increasing oral intake by allowing flexibility in the type, quantity and timing of meals.[43] Encouraging Adrian and Christie to make meal times as enjoyable as possible may also be helpful.

However, while studies that have compared nutritional counseling and/ or commercial oral liquid supplements with various control interventions for patients with cancer generally report improved caloric intake, they do not report improvements in nutritional status overall.[43] Moreover, studies of patients with advanced cancer generally report no differences in progressive weight loss in patients who received nutritional counseling and liquid oral supplementation.[44] As Adrian's disease progresses, it is important to recognize that aggressive efforts to encourage food intake may be a source of conflict and distress. Ongoing assessment of Adrian's goals of care and personal preferences and support for Christie are essential to avoid such problems.

## References

1 Dodd M, Janson, S., Facione N, *et al.* Advancing the science of symptom management. *J Adv Nurs.* 2001; **33**: 668–76.

2 Caroci Ade S, Lareau SC. Descriptors of dyspnea by patients with chronic obstructive pulmonary disease versus congestive heart failure. *Heart Lung.* 2004; **33**: 102–10.

3 Krishnasamy M. Fatigue in advanced cancer – meaning before measurement? *Int J Nurs Stud.* 2000; **37**: 401–14.

4 O'Leary U. Psychosocial influences on pain perceptions in cancer. *Nurs Times.* 2002; **98**: 36–8.

5 Queensland University of Technology. *Palliative care: a learning resource for undergraduate students.* Brisbane: Australian Department of Health and Ageing; 2005.

6 Foley K, Foley K. Pain assessment and cancer pain syndromes. Chapter 9.2.2. In: Doyle D, Hanks G, MacDonald N, eds. *Oxford Textbook of Palliative Medicine.* 2nd ed. Oxford: Oxford University Press; 1998.

7 World Health Organization. Cancer pain relief: with a guide to opioid availability. 2nd ed. Geneva: WHO; 1996.

8 Jadad A, Bowman G. The WHO analgesic ladder for cancer pain management. *JAMA* 1995; **274**: 1870–3.

9 Hanks GW, Conno F, Cherny N, *et al.* Morphine and alternative opioids in cancer pain: the EAPC recommendations. *Br J Cancer.* 2001 Mar 2; **84**(5): 587–93.

10 Cherny N, Ripamonti C, Pereira J, *et al.* Strategies to manage the adverse effects of oral morphine: an evidence-based report. *J Clin Oncol.* 2001 May 1; **19**(9): 2542–54.

11 McNicol E, Strassels S, Goudas L, *et al.* Nonsteroidal anti-inflammatory drugs, alone or combined with opioids, for cancer pain: a systematic review. *J Clin Oncol.* 2004 May 15; **22**(10): 1975–92.

12 McQuay HJ, Collins SL, Carroll D, *et al.* Radiotherapy for the palliation of painful bone metastases. *Cochrane Database of Systematic Reviews.* 1999; Issue 3.

13 Ross JR, Saunders Y, Edmonds PM, *et al.* A systematic review of the role of bisphosphonates in metastatic disease. *Health Technol Assess.* 2004; **8**(4): 1–176.

14 Wong R, Wiffen PJ. Bisphosphonates for the relief of pain secondary to bone metastases. *Cochrane Database of Systematic Reviews.* 2002; Issue 2.

15 McQuay HJ, Tramer M, Nye BA, *et al.* A systematic review of antidepressants in neuropathic pain. *Pain.* 1996 Dec; **68**(2–3): 217–27.

16 Wiffen P, Collins S, McQuay H, *et al.* Anticonvulsant drugs for acute and chronic pain. *Cochrane Database of Systematic Reviews.* 2005; Issue 2.

17 Spross J, Wolfe-Burke M. Non pharmocologic management of cancer pain. In: McGuire D, Yarbro C, Ferrell B, editors. *Cancer pain management.* 2nd ed. Boston: Jones & Bartlett; 1995.

18 Fellowes D, Barnes K, Wilkinson S. Aromatherapy and massage for symptom relief in patients with cancer. *Cochrane Database of Systematic Reviews.* 2004; Issue 3.

19 Devine EC. Meta-analysis of the effect of psychoeducational interventions on pain in adults with cancer. *Oncol Nurs Forum.* 2003; **30**: 75–89.

20 Deng G, Cassileth BR. Integrative oncology: complementary therapies for pain, anxiety, and mood disturbance. *CA Cancer J Clin.* 2005 Mar–Apr; **55**(2): 109–16.

21 Glare P, Pereira G, Kristjanson LJ, *et al.* Systematic review of the efficacy of antiemetics in the treatment of nausea in patients with far-advanced cancer. *Support Care Cancer.* 2004 Jun; **12**(6): 432–40.

22 Body J, Mancini I. Bisphosphonates for cancer patients: why, how, and when? *Support Care Cancer.* 2002; **10**: 399–407.

23 Gralla RJ, Osoba D, Kris MG, *et al.* Recommendations for the use of antiemetics: evidence-based, clinical practice guidelines. American Society of Clinical Oncology. *J Clin Oncol.* 1999 Sep; **17**(9): 2971–94.

24 Rhodes VA, McDaniel RA. Nausea, vomiting, and retching: complex problems in palliative care. *CA Cancer J Clin.* 2001; **51**: 232–48.

25 Mundy EA, DuHamel KN, Montgomery GH. The efficacy of behavioral interventions for cancer treatment-related side effects. *Semin Clin Neuropsychiatry.* 2003; **8**: 253–75.

26 Pan CX, Morrison RS, Ness J, *et al.* Complementary and alternative medicine in the management of pain, dyspnea, and nausea and vomiting near the end of life: a systematic review. *J Pain Sympt Manage.* 2000; **20**: 374–87.

27 Jennings AL, Davies AN, Higgins JPT, *et al.* Opioids for the palliation of breathlessness in terminal illness. *Cochrane Database of Systematic Reviews.* 2001; Issue 3.

28 Breslin E. The pattern of respiratory muscle recruitment during pursed-lip breathing. *Chest.* 1992; **101**: 75–8.

29 Vitacca M, Clini E, Bianchi L, *et al.* Acute effects of deep diaphragmatic breathing in COPD patients with chronic respiratory insufficiency. *Eur Respir J.* 1998; **11**: 408–15.

30 Bredin M, Corner J, Krishnasamy M, *et al.* Multicentre randomised controlled trial of nursing intervention for breathlessness in patients with lung cancer. *BMJ* 1999; **318**: 901–4.

31 Hately J, Laurence V, Scott A, *et al.* Breathlessness clinics within specialist palliative care settings can improve the quality of life and functional capacity of patients with lung cancer. *Palliat Med.* 2003; **17**: 410–7.

32 Corner J, Plant H, A'Hern R, *et al.* Non-pharmacological intervention for breathlessness in lung cancer. *Palliat Med.* 1996; **10**: 299–305.

33 Edmonds P. Is the presence of dyspnea a risk factor for morbidity in cancer patients? *J Pain Sympt Manage.* 2000; **19**: 15–22.

34 Thompson E, Sola I, Subirana M. Non-invasive interventions for improving well-being and quality of life in patients with lung cancer – a systematic review of the evidence. *Lung Cancer.* 2005; **50**: 163–7.

35 Johnson M, Moore S. Research into practice: the reality of implementing a non-pharmacological breathlessness intervention into clinical practice. *Eur J Oncol Nurs.* 2003; **7**: 33–8.

36 Rozans M, Dreisbach A, Lertora JJ, *et al.* Palliative uses of methylphenidate in patients with cancer: a review. *J Clin Oncol.* 2002 Jan 1; **20**(1): 335–9.

37 Van der Lee ML, Van der Bom JG, Swarte NB, *et al.* Euthanasia and depression: a prospective cohort study among terminally ill cancer patients. *J Clin Oncol.* 2005 Sep 20; **23**(27): 6607–12.

38  Stevinson C, Lawlor D, Fox K. Exercise interventions for cancer patients: systematic review of controlled trials. *Cancer Causes Control.* 2004; **15**: 1035–56.

39  Headley JA, Ownby KK, John LD. The effect of seated exercise on fatigue and quality of life in women with advanced breast cancer. *Oncol Nurs Forum.* 2004 Sep; **31**(5): 977–83.

40  Clark P, Lacasse C. Cancer related fatigue: clinical practice issues. *Cl J Oncol Nurs.* 1998; 2: 45–54.

41  Cimprich B. Developing an intervention to restore attention in cancer patients. *Cancer Nurs.* 1993; **16**: 83–92.

42  Loprinzi CL, Kugler JW, Sloan JA, *et al.* Randomized comparison of megestrol acetate versus dexamethasone versus fluoxymesterone for the treatment of cancer anorexia/ cachexia. *J Clin Oncol.* 1999 Oct; **17**(10): 3299–306.

43  Inui A. Cancer anorexia-cachexia syndrome: current issues in research and management. *CA Cancer J Clin.* 2002; **52**: 72–91.

44  Brown J. A systematic review of the evidence on symptom management of cancer-related anorexia and cachexia. *Oncol Nurs Forum.* 2002; **29**: 517–32.

# CHAPTER 7

# Enhancing the patient–clinician relationship

*GEOFFREY MITCHELL, STEPHEN BARCLAY*

## Introduction

According to Burge, the median length of time an individual attends a family or general practitioner is 12 years (F Burge, personal communication). This long relationship brings many benefits. For the doctor, there is the knowledge of the person's physical, psychological and social profile. The depth to which the doctor can know the patient is staggering. For the patient, the relationship leads to a level of trust and respect unattainable with other professionals they encounter in everyday life. For both, there is the likelihood that a close and unique bond will develop: friendship, but in a professional setting.

Steinhauser asked patients and carers what care would contribute to a 'good death'. Six main themes emerged: good pain and symptom management, clear decision-making, preparation for death, a sense of completion of life tasks, contributing to others, and affirmation by the care of the whole person.[1] This unique relationship between patient and GP should make the attainment of these goals possible.

The GP is in an excellent position to have a major role in the care of people when their time to die arrives. He or she will know the course of the illness, and the patient's and close family's likely response to it. This knowledge, if accessed by specialists involved, should make a significant contribution to the nature of the care the patient receives. Once the care has started, GPs should be in a position to contribute to the patient's care positively. They should have sound knowledge of the pathophysiology of the condition, sound understanding of the treatments on offer, and the ability to administer many of these. They will be able to visit the patient at home when the illness becomes too severe for office visits. Importantly, they have the ongoing contact with the surviving carers to ensure that bereavement proceeds appropriately.

All of these characteristics of primary medical care should lead to an enhancement of the relationship between the patient, the GP, the carers and the palliative care team during the course of a life-limiting illness. This chapter explores the many facets of this relationship, including the role of the GP as patient advocate and, potentially team leader. It highlights the important role of interpreting complex medical concepts, and of assisting the patient to navigate an often complex health care system. It concludes by examining the forces that threaten to undermine the value of the relationship.

In this chapter we will use the real case of Tom Hargraves, a patient of Dr Barclay's, who died at the age of 21 from malignant melanoma. Tom's story was presented at a medical grand round at Addenbrooke Hospital, Cambridge, England, by Dr Barclay, Tom's parents Allan and Annie, and Dr Pippa Corrie, his oncologist.

## The scope of palliative care in general practice

Most patients who have a life-limiting illness die in some form of institution, but 90% of the last year of life is spent at home under the care of a GP.[2] Frequently, domiciliary nurses are involved in the care as well. GPs' exposure to palliative care is small but consistent. Ninety-four percent of Canadian GPs cared for at least one dying patient at home during the previous two years,[3] and Australian GPs see a mean of five to six terminally ill patients per annum.[4] In two years, family doctors in the UK refer a mean of 5.5 terminally ill patients to specialist inpatient palliative care services, a further 4.7 patients to specialist palliative home care teams, and care for two patients without any input from specialist palliative care services.[5] Although GPs provide much of the medical care, domiciliary nurses see the patient far more frequently.[6]

Care at home – and possibly dying at home – are very important goals for patients. Patients state a preference for management by the GP and a wish to die at home.[7] While this may not always be feasible or possible, it is what most patients and carers aspire to at the outset of the palliative care journey. The increasing burden of care that carers experience leads to a change of mind with time, so that near death approximately half of people will prefer to die at home[8] compared with rates ranging from 67% to 100% if circumstances were ideal.[9–11] Curiously, broader community surveys in Australia[12] and Britain[7] expressed lower preferences – around 60% – for dying at home.

The carer, knowing the patient's preference for place of death and agreeing to it, is the main predictor for actually achieving this.[13] This was certainly the Hargraves family experience, related by his mother (*see* below). Note how the patient's preference changed in response to circumstances, and the GP's role in facilitating this.

> After the diagnosis Tom asked me to inform Stephen, our GP, who immediately arranged to visit us and to go and see Tom in hospital. He conveyed a belief that it should be possible to control Tom's symptoms so he could come home.
>
> Although Tom, and all of us, really wanted him to be at home, Tom had already chosen to stay in hospital, at least for the duration of the radiotherapy. There had been one failed and distressing attempt to treat Tom from home followed by re-admission through A & E. He didn't want to risk the pain and sickness returning, away from the relatively swift relief available in hospital.
>
> But Tom's choice was based on his difficult experience to date and he, and we, needed support and assurance to see that it really was worth trying again with a palliative care regime in place. Stephen really listened to us and encouraged us to believe that the vomiting and pain could be controlled at home. Within a short time of coming home Tom's symptoms were under reasonable control. It was a success! I won't pretend these times were easy, but we were able to be ourselves in our own place and the change in Tom's demeanour was huge! Dying in your own home is something most people want to be able to do. We are really grateful that it was made possible for Tom. (*Annie, Tom's mother*)

It is clear that the relationship between the Hargrave family and their GP was of a high caliber. When the diagnosis became apparent, they knew to call Dr Barclay. He responded promptly, and arranged calls both to the parents at home and to Tom in hospital.

## The relationship between GP and patient and carer

The principles of family practice enunciated by McWhinney[14] highlight the importance of continuity of care. The contact between the patient and GP frequently precedes the development of a disease state. The responsibility of the GP transcends a patient's age, gender or current condition. It is not terminated by the cessation of an episode of illness, or a course of treatment. In this context it is not terminated or affected by the failure to cure.

For many people their relationship with their GP stretches back a long way. For others the relationship is far more recent. The longer the relationship, the more likely it is that the GP will have developed significant understanding of the patient's context. This includes knowledge of the patient's medical history, their family and social contexts, and their personality, belief systems and likely responses to illness and pressure. GPs who have a more recent relationship with their patient will not have developed this to the same extent.

## What do patients and carers want from their GPs?

Patients and carers have certain expectations of the care their GP will provide in the context of terminal illness.

Relief of the distress from symptoms and competent medical care are clearly high priorities for patients. Devery and colleagues found from patients that the perception of the quality of medical care offered relates more to process than to outcome: the time given to patients to receive information and allow for emotions to be expressed, positive encouragement, known access to 24-hour support, and the consideration given to those around the patient as well as the patients themselves.[15] Farber and colleagues describe the features both carers and patients want from their family practitioner: primarily clinical competence, as well as a sense that the practitioner is hearing their concerns and showing more care than would normally be expected (e.g. unscheduled phone calls, home visits).[16]

Annie and Alan Hargraves reported actions by Dr Barclay that were of the highest order in this context:

> *Annie:*  Tom did not find it easy to talk about his situation. So it was really important that he always had time alone with Stephen, as indeed he had with his Drs in hospital. His adult dignity was maintained.
>
> *Allan:*  And Stephen even spent some time with Tom's mates, helping them to know what to expect, how they could support Tom and what it might mean for themselves. As a result they were able to stick with Tom right through his illness and even came to sit with his body after he'd died – not easy for four awkward 21 year olds!

In Canada, advanced cancer patients who had a continuing relationship with a GP were 1.5 times more likely to die out of hospital[17] and 3.9 times less likely to visit an emergency room.[18]

## The GP's clinical performance as reported by primary carers

The adequacy of the physical care of the individual is critically important for carers. Carers rate the distress of patients' symptoms more highly than the patients do themselves.[19] The performance of GPs in controlling pain and other symptoms is somewhat worse than practitioners caring for patients in inpatient units.[20] A 1990 national survey in the UK of the relatives of people who had died of cancer showed that at some stage in the last year of life, 88% were reported to have been in pain and 66% were said to have found it to be 'very distressing'.

Treatment that only partially controlled the pain, or not at all, was reported to have been received by 47% of those treated for pain by their GPs and by 35% of hospital patients. Seale and Cartwright found that 67% of dying patients without cancer complained of pain in the last year of life.[21] Busse *et al.* in Germany reported 100% of 47 terminally ill patients cared for at home complained of pain in the last week of life, with satisfactory control in 57% of cases.[22]

In spite of these concerning figures, the care offered by GPs was rated well by patients.[23–27] Carers considered the performance of GPs most acceptable when they enhanced the ease of getting an appointment, were willing to make home visits, took time to listen and discuss matters fully, and made efforts regarding symptom relief.[26] Farber *et al.* in the USA described these qualities as well, adding the appreciation of doctors' actions that were beyond the normal expectations of medical care (e.g. helping a patient to the car).[16] Grande *et al.*'s study in Britain confirmed the critical importance of ready access to nursing and medical care.[28] They found that many GPs were prepared to go to significant lengths to make themselves available. Many bereaved carers reported appreciation of the caring attitude of GPs and district nurses. These qualities eclipsed symptom control in importance in a study where the carers were not prompted to comment on this or other specific aspects of care.

In the eyes of bereaved carers in the UK, patients of GPs working alone experienced worse care than those of teams involving a nurse specialist, GP and district nurse, which provided the best services for patients who required symptom relief.[29] Causes of dissatisfaction noted by relatives centered around deficiencies of communication.[30] In Australia, similar interviews of carers six weeks after the death of the person cared for showed appreciation of the care provided by the palliative care team involved and the patient's GP. However, there were GPs whose care was disappointing. Nine carers out of 65 changed GPs as a result of the care they received. The issues that were important were the same: accessibility, doing home visits and being seen to make attempts to overcome symptoms.[31]

## Teamwork

Some outcomes for patients have been shown to improve when GPs and specialists teams work in collaboration. GP participation in palliative care teams has been shown to result in improved diagnostic accuracy,[32] application of evidence-based treatments,[33] identification of systematic problems in the delivery of care,[34] and improved ability to facilitate deaths at home.[35] By contrast, a trial of a consultation-only palliative care service in San Francisco[36,37] utilized a model where recommendations from the consultation service were passed on to primary care providers (PCPs) after their assessment. It was the PCPs who had the responsibility of putting them into action. The trial showed improvements in dyspnea and anxiety, improved sleep quality and spiritual well-being (i.e. conditions where the specialist team had some direct input into management). However, there were no changes in pain control or depression (where recommendation to PCPs was the only input). The authors found that PCPs did not act on many recommendations, particularly for prescriptions for analgesia and antidepressants.

Why is this? Could it be that engagement by the palliative team of primary care professionals beyond simply offering opinions or recommendations is necessary to bring out the best in them? Can intersectoral communication work in the opposite direction and contribute to improved specialist care? A trial of teleconferenced case conferences in Australia certainly suggests there may be benefits in routine direct interaction between the two groups.[38] Although they were not easy to organize, there is clear evidence that they were appreciated by the GPs as one of the few ways they could talk directly with specialist team members. The specialist teams found them useful as a way of assessing the GP's knowledge of the patient, their knowledge of palliative medicine treatments, and their willingness and ability to conduct home care. The team also recognized the potential of these virtual meetings to provide education on a range of skills pertinent to palliative care provision. However, teamwork required effort on the part of every member to maintain.

Intersectoral co-operation was also tested in the UK, where a trial of 'hospital at home' was conducted.[39] A randomized trial of hospital in the home (intensive home nursing support and medical care delivered by GPs) could not show an influence for place of death for palliative care patients in the community. However, it did make a difference to the need to call out GPs for emergency care, reduced anxiety and depression in patients as perceived by the patient's GPs, as well as improving access to out-of-hours care and some perceived improvement of symptoms.[40]

Patients cared for by teams of practitioners have better outcomes than those cared for by the GP alone.[29] This may be due to the differing perspectives on the patient's problems each professional brings. Grande et al. have identified that GPs frequently fail to identify the symptoms they find difficult to manage and those seen less commonly.[32] Moreover, domiciliary nurses in this study sought out conditions they could manage and missed those they could not. These symptoms were different from those the GPs identified.

It goes without saying that the patient and the carers are integral members of the team. One of the main issues for patients as they become more ill is the loss of control they experience as their physical capacity to function diminishes (this is discussed at length in Chapter 4). Therefore, whatever the GP and the team can do to help the retention of control will be valued. Treatment options should be discussed and the opinion of the patient gained. Another technique is to ensure that the language we use as professionals is as clear and unambiguous as possible. Euphemisms may be used to soften the message, but may also confuse and frighten:

Allan:    We were aware, from an early stage, that Tom's case was unusual and interesting from a medical perspective. It didn't happen often, but there were glimpses, occasionally, of a look which said: 'Gosh, what an unusual presentation. How interesting!' And language. All of us in the family were exposed to a vocabulary which was new to us.

Annie:    Words, which mean one thing to you, may mean something quite different to your patients. What for you is familiar technical vocabulary may be slicing into our souls, stirring up all sorts of pain in those you're talking to. You can't avoid it but be aware it may be happening.

Pippa:    Doctors are human beings: we don't always get it right. But we need to be ourselves, say and do the things that come naturally to us: don't be tempted to be defensive and hide behind technobabble; think what it would be like to be on the receiving end of some of the conversations we have; 'cancer progression', 'new growth',' seedlings', 'harvesting' . . . positive words in every day use associated with a very different picture in oncology. Be honest, always tell the truth with compassion, reach out and make physical contact, don't be afraid to cry with your patient. Our errors are easily forgiven by patients and families who sense that we really care.

Tom's care was clearly a team effort. At the outset, Dr Barclay consulted with the oncologist Dr Corrie about the likely treatment options open to him. Both in the hospital and at home, a string of professionals were involved. In spite of this, there was a sense of cohesion and purpose that resulted in the family feeling confident in the care offered.

Allan:    There were many different medical faces over those months. Our GP, Pippa and her oncology team, neurologists, surgeons, radiologists, receptionists, community nurses, pain control specialists, physiotherapist and a Marie Curie nurse, and a host of others behind the scenes whom we never met. However, we did not experience Tom's care as fragmented. There was continuity of familiar faces and a sense of a multidisciplinary partnership – communicating with each other and with us, all with Tom's best interests at heart.

Dr Barclay:    Palliative care at home is very much a partnership with the family and lay carers.

## The impact of palliative care on the GP

The care of palliative care patients encapsulates all facets of good general practice: if a GP does palliative care well, he or she will do general practice well. However, while palliative care can be relatively straightforward, problems arise that are beyond the skill of a generalist. Now that palliative care specialist teams exist, there is backup advice and support for most GPs.

However, having those teams available in most locations is not a reason to cede all palliative care to them. There are too many people who will die, and specialist teams cannot cope with them all. It is in everyone's interest for GPs to be competent at it. Routine training in palliative care has not always been readily available, a situation that has improved considerably in recent years. For example, M and F Lloyd-Williams in 1996 reported that only 15% of recently graduated UK trainees had received tutorials on palliative care from within their practice. Less than a third felt they had received adequate teaching on pain and symptom control, and fewer than 10% perceived the teaching on psychological support to be adequate. Older GPs reported learning it on the job.[41] They reported in 2003 that only 5% of 240 training schemes had no palliative care component, but the content and experience offered differed substantially. In the UK, all medical schools provide some palliative care training, frequently integrated into other parts of the curriculum.[42]

The length of time spent in general practice is the best predictor of comfort in palliative care management.[43] Not surprisingly, therefore, experience predicts the level of involvement of GPs in palliative care.[44] GPs who do participate describe the experience as a privilege.[45]

Finally, it is worth considering the costs to GPs doing palliative care. Most GPs are prepared to bear the burden of extra home visits, and possible night calls for their own patients. Palliative care is not financially rewarded as well as most other medical services. Most GPs find the communication and interpersonal conflicts often encountered in affected families difficult – in fact more so than the physical symptoms. They can feel the loss of patients, particularly long-standing ones, keenly. There may be patients GPs feel particularly sensitive to – the young, people the same age as the GP, or close family members.

> *Stephen:* Looking after Tom was emotionally the hardest task I have had since I qualified, if also deeply rewarding. The family took me inside their circle of love and care, and his death was a real bereavement to me. My DN colleagues and I found his funeral an important opportunity to say goodbye.

## Threats to GP participation in palliative care

There are significant structural barriers becoming apparent in the general practice workforce, which are likely to affect the way palliative care is practiced in the near future. They create barriers to GP involvement.

The main one is a change in attitude of younger graduates to the lifestyle taken for granted in clinical medicine. Younger graduates are much less likely to work excessively long hours to the exclusion of a life outside of clinical practice. More are likely to be female and to have competing childcare priorities, more are working part time and living considerable distances from their place of work. They are less likely to do home visits because of security concerns, particularly out of hours. Since accessibility and the ability and willingness to do home visits are important prerequisites of care from the primary carer point of view, it is likely that the care offered will be by fewer people willing to do it, probably older practitioners, with relatively few new people prepared to take it on. More will fall to the specialist services, who may not be able to cope.[46]

In addition, because length of time in practice is a predictor of comfort in palliative care, getting started involves significant departures from clinical comfort – another disincentive for young practitioners to get involved. There is a temptation on behalf of some specialists to simply pick up the load and not try to engage the GP.[46] This strategy will only perpetuate the problem.

Finally, the wider structures of clinical practice, with a move towards after-hours co-operatives or triage services not staffed by clinicians with any contact with the patient's practice, is leading to a situation of reduced continuity of care becoming commonplace. This will have adverse consequences for patients, because the after-hours practitioners are likely not to have been provided with information about the patient's condition.[47] On the other hand, the palliative care framework devised by Thomas has been embraced by approximately a third of UK practices. It sets benchmarks for palliative care service delivery which, if implemented widely, will lead to practices delivering effective palliative care.[48]

A range of strategies on the part of government and palliative care specialist services will be required to encourage young GPs to start practicing palliative care, make allowances for the non-medical demands on their lives, and at the same time ensure no patient is disadvantaged by care models that don't meet their needs.[46] If they can be encouraged to start, there is a chance they will reach the point where they become comfortable with the care of dying patients.

## References

1 Steinhauser K, Clipp EC, McNeilly M, *et al*. In search of a good death: observations of patients, families, and providers. *Ann Int Med*. 2000; **132**: 825–32.
2 Hinton J. Can home care maintain an acceptable quality of life for patients with terminal cancer and their relatives? *Palliat Med*. 1994; **8**: 183–96.

3 McWhinney IR. Caring for patients with cancer: family physicians' role. *Can Fam Physician.* 1994; **40**: 16–19.

4 Wakefield MA, Beilby J, Ashby MA. General practitioners and palliative care. *Palliat Med.* 1993; **7**: 117–26.

5 Higginson I. Palliative care services in the community: what do family doctors want? *J Palliat Care.* 1999; **15**: 21–5.

6 Hinton J. Services given and help perceived during home care for terminal cancer. *Palliat Med.* 1996; **10**(2): 125–34.

7 Charlton RC. Attitudes towards care of the dying: a questionnaire survey of general practice attenders. *Fam Pract.* 1991; **8**: 356–9.

8 Higginson IJ, Sen-Gupta GJ. Place of care in advanced cancer: a qualitative systematic literature review of patient preferences. *J Palliat Med.* 2000; **3**: 287–300.

9 Townsend J, Frank AO, Fermont D, *et al.* Terminal cancer care and patients' preference for place of death: a prospective study. *BMJ* 1990; **301**: 415–17.

10 Dunlop R, Davies R, Hockley H. Preferred versus actual place of death: a hospital palliative care support team experience. *Palliat Med.* 1989; **3**: 197–201.

11 Tiernan E, O'Connor M, O'Siorain L, *et al.* A prospective study of preferred versus actual place of death among patients referred to a palliative care home-care service. *Ir Med J.* 2002; **95**: 232–5.

12 Ashby M, Wakefield M. Attitudes to some aspects of death and dying, living wills and substituted health care decision-making in South Australia: public opinion survey for a parliamentary select committee. *Palliat Med.* 1993; **7**: 273–82.

13 Cantwell P, Turco S, Brenneis C, *et al.* Predictors of home death in palliative care cancer patients. *J Palliat Care.* 2000; **16**: 23–8.

14 McWhinney IR. Principles of family medicine. In: McWhinney IR. *A Textbook of Family Medicine.* New York: Oxford University Press; 1997.

15 Devery K, Lennie I, Cooney N. Health outcomes for people who use palliative care services. *J Palliat Care.* 1999; **15**: 5–12.

16 Farber S, Egnew T, Herman-Bertsch J, *et al.* Issues in end-of-life care: patient, caregiver, and clinician perceptions. *J Palliat Med.* 2003; **6**: 19–31.

17 Burge F, Lawson B, Johnston G, *et al.* Primary care continuity and location of death for those with cancer. *J Palliat Med.* 2003; **6**: 911–18.

18 Burge F, Lawson B, Johnston G. Family physician continuity of care and emergency department use in end-of-life cancer care. *Med Care.* 2003; **41**: 992–1001.

19 Field D, Douglas C, Jagger C, *et al.* Terminal illness: views of patients and their lay carers. *Palliat Med.* 1995; **9**: 45–54.

20 Addington Hall J, McCarthy M. Dying from cancer: results of a national population-based investigation. *Palliat Med.* 1995; **9**: 295–305.

21 Seale C, Cartwright. A. *The Year Before Death.* Oxford: Oxford University Press; 1994.

22 Busse R, Wagner HP, Krauth C, *et al.* Sentinel practices in evaluating longer periods of care: quality of life and drug therapy of terminally ill persons in Lower Saxony (Germany). *J Epidemiol Community Health.* 1998; **52**: 156s–60s.

23 Addington-Hall J, McCarthy M. Dying from cancer: results of a national population-based investigation. *Palliat Med.* 1995; **9**: 295–305.

24 Higginson I, Wade A, McCarthy M. Palliative care: views of patients and their families. *BMJ* 1990; **301**: 277–81.

25 Holden J, Brindley J, O'Donnell S, *et al.* An audit of 319 deaths across four general practices. *Br J Clin Pract.* 1996; **50**: 79–80.

26 Lecouturier J, Jacoby A, Bradshaw C, *et al.* Lay carer's satisfaction with community palliative care: results of a postal survey. *Palliat Med.* 1999; **13**: 275–83.

27 Hanratty B. Palliative care provided by GPs: the carer's viewpoint. *Br J Gen Pract.* 2000; **50**: 653–4.

28 Grande G, Farquhar M, Barclay SIG, *et al.* Valued aspects of primary palliative care: content analysis of bereaved carers' descriptions. *Br J Gen Pract.* 2004; **54**: 772–8.

29 Hearn J, Higginson I. Do specialist palliative care teams improve outcomes for cancer patients?: a systematic literature review. *Palliat Med.* 1998; **12**: 317–32.

30 Blyth AC. Audit of terminal care in a general practice. *BMJ* 1990; **300**: 983–6.

31 Mitchell G. The effect of case conferences between general practitioners and palliative care specialist teams on the quality of life of dying people. [PhD]. Brisbane: University of Queensland; 2005.

32 Grande GE, Barclay SI, Todd CJ. Difficulty of symptom control and general practitioners' knowledge of patients' symptoms. *Palliat Med.* 1997; **11**: 399–406.

33 Mitchell G. Assessment of GP management of symptoms of dying patients in an Australian community hospice by chart audit. *Fam Pract.* 1998; **15**: 420–5.

34 Robinson L, Stacy R. Palliative care guidelines in the community: setting practice guidelines for primary care teams. *Br J Gen Pract.* 1994; **44**: 461–4.

35 Costantini M, Camoirano E, Madeddu L, *et al.* Palliative home care and place of death among cancer patients: a population-based study. *Palliat Med.* 1993; **7**: 323–31.

36 Rabow M, Petersen J, Schanche K, *et al.* The comprehensive care team: a description of a controlled trial of care at the beginning of the end of life. *J Palliat Med.* 2003; **6**: 489–99.

37 Rabow M, Dibble S, Panitlat S, *et al.* The comprehensive care team: a controlled trial of outpatient palliative medicine consultation. *Arch Int Med.* 2004; **164**: 83–91.

38 Mitchell G, Cherry M, Kennedy R, *et al.* General practitioner–specialist providers case conferences in palliative care: lessons learned from 56 case conferences. *Aust Fam Physician.* 2005; **34**: 389–92.

39 Grande G, Todd C, Barclay S, *et al.* Does hospital at home of palliative care facilitate death at home?: a randomised controlled trial. *BMJ* 1999; **319**: 1472–5.

40 Grande GE, Todd CJ, Barclay SI, *et al.* A randomized controlled trial of a hospital at home service for the terminally ill. *Palliat Med.* 2000; **14**: 375–85.

41 Lloyd Williams M, Lloyd Williams F. Palliative care teaching and today's general practitioners: is it adequate? *Eur J Cancer Care (Engl).* 1996; **5**: 242–5.

42 Field D, Wee B. Preparation for palliative care: teaching about death, dying and bereavement in UK medical schools 2000–2001. *Med Educ.* 2002; **36**: 561–7.

43 Lopez de Maturana A, Morago V, San Emeterio E, *et al.* Attitudes of general practitioners in Bizkaia, Spain, towards the terminally ill patient. *Palliat Med.* 1993; **7**: 39–45.

44 Hunt RW, Radford AJ, Maddocks I, *et al.* The community care of terminally ill patients. *Aust Fam Physician.* 1990; **19**: 1835–41.

45 Field D. Special not different: general practitioners' accounts of their care of dying people. *Soc Sci Med.* 1998; **46**: 1111–20.

46 Reymond E, Mitchell G, McGrath B, *et al. Research into the Educational, Training and Support Needs of General Practitioners in Palliative Care: report to the Commonwealth of Australia.* Brisbane: Mt Olivet Health Services; 2003.

47 Burt J, Shipman C, Barclay S, *et al*. Continuity within primary palliative care: an audit of general practice out-of-hours co-operatives. *J Public Health (Oxf)*. 2004; **26**: 275–6.

48 Thomas K. In search of a good death: primary healthcare teams work in new framework for better care of the dying at home. *BMJ* 2003; **327**: 223.

# CHAPTER 8

# Health promotion and palliative care

*ALLAN KELLEHEAR*

## Introduction

An important element of the patient-centered model is that of health promotion. For the most part, this implies that the family doctor utilizes opportunities afforded by the patient presenting themselves to explore one or more health issues which may prevent illness in the long term. The idea that health promotion has a place in the context of palliative care seems contradictory. Surely in a dying patient, there is no room for preventive advice?

Allan Kellehear explores this seemingly contradictory juxtaposition in this chapter and he shows that a literal reading of the principles of health promotion provides ample scope for their application in a palliative care setting.

## Health promotion in palliative care?

Health promotion and palliative care often look like strange companions, if not mismatched buddies. Although we are accustomed to thinking about health promotion in relation to sexual health, workplace safety or diabetes education, we frequently do not associate these health promotion ideas and practices with palliative care. We commonly view palliative care as 'terminal care', or at the very least as care for people in the last weeks or months of life. But that is only part of the historical and practice story of palliative care, and really only the part of palliative care that is most popularly understood. In this way, health-promoting palliative care is less recognized and therefore can sometimes appear counter-intuitive.

However, in some form or another, palliative care has always extended beyond this narrow stereotype of its 'terminal' care image. Because palliative care is, like most medicine, holistic care – care of the social, spiritual and psychological aspects of a person and not just people's bodies alone – it also embraces a palliative approach. Palliative care is not only whole-person care, but specifically whole-person care of anyone with a life-threatening illness for which there is no cure. Managing the physical symptoms of a life-threatening illness is certainly crucial to that care, but the task of keeping them as well as possible is also important. So clinical treatments are partnered with broader but no less important care plans that include supporting good personal morale (psychology), social support (family and other social networks), and meaning-making (spiritual and pastoral care).

These care plans do not (and should not) occur in a vacuum, and so are not without some basic underpinning ideas. To start with, good health has as its foundation the physical and social context of life. In other words, our everyday cycles of work and play occur in a physical and social environment that plays a crucial determinant in our health and illness outcomes. In this way, poor sources of drinking-water, a lack of sexual health knowledge, or communities built near flood plains or drought-prone areas are just as important predictors of an individual's health risk as an individual's genetics.

We have always known about this intimate relationship between social context/environment and health whenever medicine has been at the forefront of battling infectious diseases, or the rate of lung cancer in the community, or the patterned rate and type of injuries we see in our accident and emergency departments. In this way, medical science is a social science. Its practitioners have always instinctively understood that our acute care models are designed to get people out of trouble and our public health models are designed to prevent us from getting into trouble in the first place. Medical practice is always community practice in the bigger picture of health and illness in society.

However, it is important to recognize that when we speak about 'public health', or 'society', or indeed 'distal context', that in fact we are *not* talking about something 'out there'. Public health and society are 'in-the-head' experiences for everyone. Our personal, individual values, attitudes and conduct, and what commonly seem to be idiosyncratic affinities, social preferences or sense of esthetics, are frequently shaped, and are continually being shaped, by our interaction with others, such as colleagues, family, friends or what we read or see in newspapers or television. 'Society' is an intimate idea, an intimate personal experience for us all. This makes health promotion an experience that has personal meaning and life, as well as a more abstract existence in the form of changes in health legislation or the publicizing of health promotion messages on our electronic airwaves.

The idea of modern health, then, is the challenge of working with the notion that health is far more than the absence of disease. In a technical sense, few of us are really disease-free. Most adults display signs of atherosclerosis, arthritis or minor episodic events such as colds or flu, for example. Few, if any of us, get through a day without minor pain or discomfort, mentally or physically. The idea of health as 'freedom from disease' is an ideological artefact of an earlier, less sophisticated view of health. Today, we accept that sound public health policy and personal health promotion are about a balance between quality health services provision and sound health promotion in the community by all of us – health services, schools, local government authorities and workplaces. We all play our part. Apart from any other consideration, such complementary understanding of public health and acute care interventions fosters seamless care across the course of the life of any disease and, of course, across our lives in general. Living with a life-threatening illness is no exception to this rule.

All these above preliminary remarks underline three common misconceptions about health promotion in general and health promotion in palliative care in particular. These misconceptions are:

▶ health promotion has little or no role to play in the shadow of death and dying
▶ health promotion is an abstract and broad set of initiatives with few practice suggestions for the individual health and medical practitioner
▶ what little practice suggestions exist merely cover what might be better and more simply understood as 'health education'.

In this chapter I would like to challenge each of these misconceptions while at the same time offering a set of practical suggestions and insights into health promotion initiatives for the lone practitioner. What, then, are the basic ideas of health promotion in palliative care?

## Central ideas of health-promoting palliative care

Health promotion is a particular style of public health practice.[1,2] Sometimes called the 'new public health,' health promotion places the emphasis on creating 'healthy' environments, keeping people healthy and applying the 'old' public health ideas of prevention and harm reduction to lifestyles rather than simply disease outbreaks.[3] Whether in private practice, as part of a broader health service, or from the point of view of bureaucrats developing policy, there are always five fundamental public health ideas when caring for people with life-threatening illness: prevention, harm reduction, community participation, health and death education, and social supports.

These five public health ideas are *not* difficult ideas, and excepting the case of death education, are the bases of all major worldwide health promotion campaigns. These ideas are worth trying to remember because they not only supply a simple philosophy about why we do the things we do in health promotion, but also why specific practice directions take the shape they so often do.

## Prevention and harm reduction

The simple idea behind the term 'prevention' is that we try to avoid the events and experiences that cause us harm. In general public health terms, for example, prevention efforts can be illustrated in the practice of avoiding excessive UV radiation, and early screening to lower rates of skin cancer. Introducing legislation to outlaw the use of asbestos in building materials also helps avoid asbestosis and other respiratory disorders. Using condoms is a front-line defence against HIV and other sexually transmissible diseases.

Another example that encompasses prevention but also harm reduction is the example of vehicle seat restraints. Seat belts both prevent and reduce harms associated with people being jettisoned from cars during a collision. Seat belts thereby substantially help us to avoid head injury or reduce the damage, avoid spinal injury or reduce the damage, or avoid death during vehicle collisions or at least substantially lower the risk of fatality.

Health promotion in palliative care is obviously not designed to prevent death, but rather the associated physical, social, psychological and spiritual problems associated with death and dying. These might include grief, depression, anxiety, hopelessness and loss of meaning, social stigma and rejection, as well as the better-known biological sequelae such as breathlessness, cachexia, and chronic or severe pain. In all these examples, some of these experiences can actually be prevented while others become targets of harm reduction.

Grief, of course, is impossible to prevent, but some of the most undesirable consequences of grief such as suicide, severe depression or serious cardiac or gastrointestinal disorders are subject to strategic harm-reduction interventions. Social stigma or rejection and hopelessness are social and spiritual experiences amenable to prevention at best, but at the very least are subject to harm-reduction strategies.

## Community participation

A crucial part of all health promotion efforts is to enlist the support of social networks that support and help sustain good health in the community. These include trade unions and school boards, particularly in matters to do with work-place safety or bullying, for example. But other less clearly defined 'communities', such as the 'gay community,' can be important to work with in promoting sexual health practices.

As we have found in HIV prevention and harm-reduction campaigns, there is little point educating an individual to use a condom when this practice is not part of the social and sexual norms of the culture where this use must occur on a regular basis. It is important to inform individuals about the harms associated with excessive use of alcohol, but it is also important to change community attitudes to drink-driving to support that individual change.

In matters to do with life-threatening illness, it is one thing to foster self-esteem in a person and quite another to sustain that attitude in the face of growing community stigma associated with HIV/AIDS, or when wearing a wig during cancer treatment. Clearly there is a complementary role to be played between individual work and community work. Individual responses are sometimes created and sometimes shaped by the social context – these are the broader interpersonal reactions, responses, attitudes or values of other people. No health promotion initiative that targets the lone individual has much chance in the wider workaday world unless that world is also part of the initiative.

## Health and death education

The most popular set of ideas associated with health promotion is the idea of 'education' – of providing people with information, personal counseling and raising public awareness. Warnings on electrical appliances or cigarette packets, explanations of how infection is spread, raising awareness about diving in unknown waters or the practice of unprotected sunbathing are all important 'education' strategies that enhance the health of populations.

As mentioned earlier, so much of health promotion has been associated with the task of 'what can I tell them?' or 'what information can I impart?' to patients and their families. Indeed, this is a crucial part of any health promotion initiative. It is important to raise awareness about grief: that it is not like the flu, and you will not necessarily 'get over it'. But grief and loss in bereavement, for example, can have some positives such as the opportunity to continue with the relationship on different grounds. Facing death or surviving the death of someone we love can be an experience of personal growth – changing attitudes, making some people more compassionate, making others great advocates of social causes, creating social, political and financial legacies for others.[4]

But grief, or stigma or meaning-making occur in a social context – in a very specific set of environments that may or may not be 'health promoting' for death and loss experiences. In this way, 'raising awareness' or 'giving information' may not be enough to withstand alternative and less constructive influences from an important social network at home, school or work.

To employ an 'old' public health example: there is little point advising individuals not to drink the polluted town water which is causing their gastro-intestinal problems when that is the *sole source* of hydration for the community. Individual education must be viewed as only one health promotion initiative in play with a concert of others. The practice problem has been that most lone practitioners have felt that patient education is the limit of their contribution, and that is not necessarily so.

## Social supports

It is clear from any observation about dying and the experience of loss that social supports are crucial to the well-being of those at the centre of these experiences. Frequently, practitioners in health have sought to assess and build on the resilience and strength of family and friends. This is particularly important in the last weeks and days of life, as well as for the first weeks and months of bereavement after the death of the patient.

However, living with a life-threatening illness can occur over much longer periods, with people living through several cycles of remission and recurrence. During these periods, supports are drawn from larger social territory, and workplaces and schools, for example, may need information and guidance to help them to provide an adequate support response to their ill co-worker or school friend. Pamphlets can be useful, as can phone calls from experienced clinicians, but sometimes only a discussion with key members of a workplace or school can help supply information, challenge myths, clarify misunderstandings and dispel fears.

Even the idea of 'support' often requires explanation or clarification. Although there are many media and clinical reports of social stigma and rejection of people with cancer, many more people report overwhelming social attention they cannot cope with.[5] This popularity attracts less attention from journalists but is no less a problem, and such well-meaning popularity can create tiredness, increased social conflict, personal guilt and stress. Most friends act as individuals and do not necessarily understand that they are or will be the 27th visitor to their sick friend's door that day.

Offering social support as a health promotion initiative is rarely as straight-forward as it might first seem, particularly in matters to do with life-threatening illness. The discussion in this section has rehearsed the key ideas behind health promotion in general as well as health promotion in palliative care. But the actual practice of these ideas requires an understanding of the requisite skills for the satisfactory expression of these ideas.

## Thinking about health promotion as a practice issue

Health promotion requires a particular style of relationship (participatory relations), targets (community and individuals, the well and the ill), and offerings (education, support and civic skills). When we think and practice health promotion, we must aspire to these as a *collection of practice offerings and targets* and avoid the temptation to slip into a one-sided paternalism or a simple didactic education approach.

### Creating participatory relations

The easiest way to summarize 'participatory relations' is to express this as 'working *with* people rather than *on* them'. Equal relations based on mutual interests but a different level and type of 'expertise' characterize the social relations of health promotion. Although a medical practitioner may have 'expert' knowledge of the harmful effects of smoking, the expertise on the environmental and personality factors that work against giving up smoking clearly resides with the smoker. Anti-smoking campaigns enjoy optimum success with *motivated* people, where the desire to give up smoking has come from those people rather than coercion from authoritative sources.

So, too, in matters to do with living with a life-threatening illness we do well to take at least some of our lead from those people rather than assuming that we know what kinds of problems they will encounter and/or how they will necessarily see or react to them. Health-promoting palliative care is fundamentally about creating a professional climate of accessibility, openness and interest in matters to do with the social, psychological and spiritual difficulties of facing death and loss. The professional literature is replete with patient stories of *not* sharing their concerns because health practitioners seemed more stressed by the topic of death than the patient!

### Educating and informing

Obviously, living with life-threatening illness requires attention to symptom control and the associated medication, clinical interventions and accessory supports. However, treatment is not about health but about the disease and its expression. We have all heard people with cancer say that there are 'good days and bad days'. And what can we do to promote, maximize or enhance the health of those with life-threatening illness on those 'good days', while reducing or minimizing any harm or stresses on those 'bad days'?

Clearly, information and a raised awareness of the pattern of health and illness in a particular disease course may be helpful. Sometimes, though, information about the process of death or dying can alleviate anxiety or outright fear. Not everyone finds the topic of death threatening, for cultural or personal reasons. People frequently have many questions about the possible manner of their own death, anxieties for survivors, fears about the afterlife, questions about purpose. Many of these can be addressed by recommending a video program, a book, or a discussion with the local pastoral care worker. Education about health in its broadest social, psychological and spiritual senses is crucial for health promotion among those living with life-threatening illness. But death education is equally important and relevant for this group and their family and friends. There is much misconception, fear and ignorance about dying, death and loss, and these are important sources of harm, discomfort and risk for many people. Death education is a vital part of any health-promoting palliative care approach.

## Targeting the well and ill

It is also important to note that working with the ill – the person with a life-threatening illness – is only one side of the health promotion equation. Many of the problems and much of the support that a person with life-threatening illness encounters are actually from others who do not have a life-threatening illness, or have never encountered death, dying or bereavement.

This broad and diverse set of publics – people inexperienced in matters of death and loss – are important targets of public health intervention, and an individual practitioner can contribute to their education by participating in public events such as radio talkback, newspaper features or school visits. Equally useful but less time consuming is the provision of poster information, reading material or video programs in the waiting room. Along with the simple messages of health promotion about fitness, controlled substance use or nutrition, people waiting to see you can learn, for example, that listening is superior to talk when it comes to supporting people in grief. Everyone benefits from a broad health-promoting palliative approach that includes those with and without life-threatening illness.

## Strengthening community action

Often health and medical practitioners are invited to participate in community activities such as community festivals or information days. At other times, health service professionals will be invited to speak at service and recreational clubs such as Rotary, Lions or the local soccer or tennis club. These are opportunities to strengthen a community's own interest in health-related matters and are important: an appearance or contribution here can be crucial to changing attitudes or encouraging helpful responses to people living with a life-threatening illness or living with loss.

Sometimes a practitioner is unable to participate in these invitations because they simply do not have the time, interest or personal resources to engage in these kinds of activities. Nevertheless, even in declining invitations to participate in a community health promotion activity, a practitioner has the opportunity to encourage organizers to include the local palliative care or grief services, services often left out – unnecessarily – from mainstream health promotion activities.

## Developing personal skills

One of the key reasons why many health and medical practitioners do not participate in civic activities, aside from time constraints, is the lack of personal skills and experience with health promotion activities such as radio talks, school visits or writing for newspapers. Apart from the lack of training in these skills, much of this problem also stems from lack of experience. But accepting some small invitations at local radio stations or volunteering to write a small column occasionally for one's regional newspaper is often gratefully accepted and is frequently supported by copy editors or experienced radio personalities. These experiences can be personally rewarding and add much to the professional and personal development of the individual practitioner, as well as being an extremely important contribution to community health.

Equally, people living with life-threatening illness sometimes need to 'skill up' for the new challenges in their life that encountering serious illness may bring. Learning to cope with change in their relationships – sexual, interpersonal or attitudinal – may mean that they will need the support of important health colleagues such as a social worker, counselor or pastoral care worker. Learning to control anxiety, even panic, during times of severe physical or treatment discomfort may mean learning new skills in relaxation control such as meditation or use of a masseur. These may require referrals to those who can assist them to learn these skills, and this may require a referral network outside the usual medical or allied health network one is accustomed to working within.

## Fostering hope

An important – indeed crucial – part of living with a life-threatening illness *and* living with loss is the delicate personal art of cultivating hope. People living with a life-threatening illness, even those with very short life expectancies, hope to have a better day tomorrow. All of us hope to maintain our connections with one another directly or indirectly over distance, over time, and often through what often seem to be the impenetrable or unknown wall we call death.

Such hopes can be fostered – and realistically fostered – through spiritual readings, joining self-help or support groups, regular conversations with a pastoral carer, old friends, or reading books about diverse religious beliefs around the world. A simple conversation about how each person living with loss or a life-threatening illness maintains his or her everyday hope is a useful conversation to have, and to have regularly. No 'screening instrument' is better than the simple question, 'How's your hope levels today?' as a routine question alongside other questions about blood sugar, blood pressure, bowel movements or nutrition. Fostering hope is an important health promotion activity for those living with serious illness and has been shown to lengthen life and increase its quality.[6–9]

## Ensuring sustainability

A final feature of all successful health promotion programs is the ability of that program to continue without your continual support of it as a health or medical practitioner. It is important that people develop an interest in their own self-care. We rely on this idea of sustainability and self-monitoring in other areas of health promotion, such as combating sedentary lifestyles or poor nutrition. People must *want* to be fit and healthy; people must *want* to eat well and take an interest in what's in the food they are eating. Otherwise health promotion programs fail or are abandoned easily, or become subject to fashion and fad.

Just as importantly, any health-promoting palliative care approach by individual practitioners must draw parallels between health and serious disease or loss, and between health and other areas of life such as driver safety or cardiovascular health. It is important that patients understand and see the value of pursuing health in these less understood areas of life-threatening illness or loss to understand that the cliché of 'quality of life' actually refers to promoting the physical, social, psychological and spiritual dimensions of all life, including those in the very shadow of death.

## Spheres of practice – what you can do

### Communication issues – diagnosis and prognostic discussion

Two personal experiences are frequently said to be similar to being 'hit by a bomb' due to their devastating and disorienting impact: being diagnosed with cancer or HIV and losing a loved one through death. Commonly, whatever is said during the first few moments, hours or days after these experiences occur is not remembered. Details of conversations with others are particularly difficult to recall. Most of us have seen this problem in many people in these situations, and so it is important that any discussion of diagnosis and prognosis occurs more than once and, initially at least, is timed soon after the first discussion of these experiences.

Whatever your communication style and whatever facial expression or personal demeanour seems to characterize the patient reaction *at the time*, it will be useful to revisit these diagnostic discussions again soon for both your sakes. Important messages of hope, comfort and problem-solving made by you at the time can be checked to see if the patient has actually heard them in the first place and repositioned by you if the patient has not understood them. After the initial shock of loss, people frequently develop a set of their own questions, and a second meeting soon after the initial one can be a crucial forum for that discussion.

A common question from people diagnosed with a cancer, HIV or similar life-threatening illness is 'How long have I got (to live)?'. Often such inquiries are insistent. It is good practice wisdom to revisit the ways we make these judgements. It is important to explain that any prognostication must be based on large epidemiological data sets of people with a similar disease, and that to attempt to grapple with the statistical unknowns of *where* an individual person might sit in that data set of possibilities and probabilities is almost impossible. This is obviously because individual genetics, character, personal attitude, and individual treatment response are not predicted by large epidemiological data sets. These 'unknowns' are some of the working materials for personal hope and positive attitude, and are important to discuss very clearly.[10,11]

## Grief and loss

Grief has a diversity of personal expression. People grieve in about as many ways as they love, the two experiences being intimately linked. The *trauma* of grief, on the other hand, has common patterns, such as sobbing fits, depression, insomnia, anger, anxiety and lack of appetite.

At a time in our society when few people speak about what serious loss means to one another, it is crucial to take some time with each person to do just that. Trauma and grief, their differences and overlaps, the negatives of grief reaction, but also the positives that frequently emerge later, are all commonly unacknowledged or misunderstood topics. Discussions about the physical effects of grief, about the problem of time or duration of certain physical or psychological reactions, and of the types and styles of help available for them are all important components of such a discussion.

Support groups, self-help groups and some types of reading or video material on grief can be very helpful. Being 'educated' about grief can be reassuring – health promoting as well as hope promoting – for people living with loss. Reading other first-person accounts of what grief is like can be helpful. Time does not heal grief, but it may torture a very traumatized person. Actively seeking help – self-help or professional help – can be health promoting and harm reducing, and a good referral network and an office well resourced with books, DVDs and videos is crucial for promoting this self-learning and social support.

## Re-education about illness

For just about every serious illness today there exists a voluntary support society (e.g. for motor neurone disease, multiple sclerosis, cancer, HIV, bereavement), and these societies are worth contacting to identify resources and people who may be useful to the newly diagnosed patients. Many of these societies practice health promotion, aiming to provide supports, education and advocacy for people with their particular medical conditions. A directory or list of such societies can be a valuable part of your information sharing with patients.

It is one thing to have an illness described by your local GP and quite another to have it described by a fellow traveler with the same diagnosis. The dock workers know where the ship is sailing, but only another passenger keeps you company during the long days and nights of the journey ahead.

Much of the practice and evaluation literature suggests that self-help groups and societies are viewed by patients as valuable resources,[12-14] but a common problem is a lack of referrals.[15] Since many of these societies run on a voluntary basis and have small budgets, advertising their services is an onerous and expensive task. Referrals in these instances become important civic tasks in health promotion by lone practitioners because they forge new alliances beyond the medical and allied health network.

## Re-education about death and dying

There is a distaste and fear surrounding discussion about death and dying. Some of this is culturally supported by a modern industrial emphasis on preferred concepts of youth, health, beauty, longevity and/or expectation of the age of retirement. Sudden death or death from life-threatening illness before the age of 90 is frequently greeted with horror. These diffuse community attitudes underwrite difficulties with talking about one's own death or dying and yet, at some point in a life-threatening illness people do frequently want to speak about these things. People become curious and develop questions about the physical process, fears about certain images of what will happen when they die, or even fears of lying in a vegetative state in a nursing home or hospital.

Other people re-examine their childhood understanding of religion, seek to understand different views – religious and research-based understandings of near-death experiences, visions or other mystical experiences. There is a wealth of reading and audio-visual material on these topics, and some discussion or guide to them can be useful. If you have spent some time examining and reflecting on some of these matters, one or two of these resources can be kept at the practice to loan out to patients or their families.

Sometimes the local grief or palliative care service may have some useful patient material on many of these and other topics, and, once again, contact can be useful health promotion work for the practice. It is always useful to have reading and watching suggestions, and although we frequently think of these things for illness groups we do not always associate them with patient education approaches to death and dying. Yet the harms from such fears, sorrows or anguish can commonly and easily be addressed with information and education, just as with any other healthcare topic. Your understanding and acknowledgement of this simple insight to a person living with loss or a life-threatening illness is itself a health- and hope-promoting message and will also assure you of a trusted place when other questions about death or dying occur to them later.

## Community participation

The most difficult challenge for an individual practitioner working alone and working long hours is to include civic participation as part of their practice – in this case, health promotion practice. There is no way to discuss this problem except plainly. If you believe that the practice of public health must have a civic component to assist with changing community attitudes to smoking, drink-driving or sexual health, or to support people with life-threatening illness or loss, some civic participation is a must.

Some readers will be content to confine their health promotion to health education and support in face-to-face encounters, but most others will argue or observe that they already participate professionally at some level in their own community for the sake of the health and safety of that community. For those readers who already do some of this work, the challenge becomes to include death and loss as part of it.

Once a year you might participate in a local service club dinner (with Lions, Apex or Rotary, for example) where you are guest speaker. Or once a year you may participate in the local community's 'fun run' as a judge or medical support person. You might give a talk at the local school or radio station. In any of these scenarios it is possible to raise awareness about grief and loss and living with a life-threatening illness. Often it is merely a question of remembering to do so because we are often asked or volunteer to chat about so many other more popular topics such as diabetes, heart health or child safety. You can foster death education in the community by integrating this topic into your interests.

Alternatively, you could contact the local palliative care or grief service to say that you are willing to help in their own health-promotion activities with the community from time to time, professional commitments permitting.

As mentioned before, the waiting room can also be used as a small group or community resource if appropriate pamphlets, books, or audio-visual material are made available there. In all these cases, we do not necessarily have to 'sell' talk. Wearing a badge about supporting carers of people with dementia or terminal illness, keeping the business cards of the local grief and bereavement service prominently on your work desk, or maintaining a diverse and interesting library of educational magazines and books within view of patients can all promote curiosity, interest, discussion and health-promoting activity in matters to do with death and loss.

## Health-promoting environments

In summary, the desire to improve the social, psychological, spiritual and physical health of those living with a life-threatening illness, or loss, and those caring for them is best accomplished, to put it in simple public health terms, by creating environments that are 'health promoting'.

There are four major practice contexts for promoting health and well-being for these people that are readily available to the lone practitioner: the direct practice context, the waiting room, the building and grounds of the practice setting, and the wider community. Each of these contexts provides important opportunities for the individual practitioner to exercise and widen his or her influence on everyone's understanding and behaviour in matters to do with death and loss.

## The direct practice context

This basic face-to-face context is the most obvious, traditional and easiest environment for practitioners to identify and work within. Here, in face-to-face interpersonal contexts, we can provide accessibility, information, education and referral. By accessibility I mean regular, closely scheduled meetings with people living with life-threatening illness or loss, but most especially those for whom this is recent news. Information can be given about diagnosis and/or prognosis, but also about maintaining health, hope and support. The need for referrals to other colleagues in medicine, allied health, complementary health or self-help and support groups can be discussed, weighed, identified and recommended.

The health-promoting style of communication in this face-to-face encounter is important to remember and foster. Encouraging talk and enquiry and facilitating the patient's own suggestions for what they might do next for themselves can be done not just by asking questions, but by spending some time discussing how they coped with troubles or bad news before – what 'worked' for them and what did not. Sometimes, your remembering and relating a story or two about what others found useful in their journey of a similar illness or bereavement can unlock their thoughts or promote creative thinking about how they might approach their own journeys.

An assurance – and evidence – of your interest in the topic of loss or death in the context of their own predicament will be important to their ability to sustain a commitment to their own health promotion and your involvement in it. Some of this 'evidence' of interest will be displayed on your desk, the books behind you, or the stories you recount to them about your own thoughts and experiences in this area.

## The waiting room

This environment should not be employed as a place 'to kill time' for people waiting to see you but as an environment that is health promoting as well as interesting. A small library can be maintained here, and among other health promotion material for heart health, diabetic health or sexual health there might also be audio-visual and reading material on death, dying, loss and care. Most relevant in this genre are books that offer first-person accounts of cancer survival, caring for those with dementia, those living with loss (especially bereavement), and popular works on the search for meaning and hope during chronic illness (for some practical reading suggestions for yourself and/or your patients, see Kellehear 1999: 77–101).[1]

Posters with simple health promotion messages are also useful. Some of these can be obtained from the local AIDS council or cancer council. Messages of support and hope for people with life-threatening illness or loss can also be made and designed with simple computer programs these days. For example, a poster might read, 'When a friend is grieving it can be more helpful to listen to them than talk at them', or 'Remember that people with serious illnesses such as cancer experience inconsistent health and need more of your understanding and support on some days than on others'. These posters or messages can change every few months.

The waiting room can also be used as a community resource for staging after-hours talks by you, your colleagues or outside associates who might provide interactive seminars or talks on topics of interest to the community in matters to do with death, dying, loss or care. Interactive computer programs, paper quizzes or crossword puzzles that explore key concepts in loss, care or life-threatening illness can also be valuable changes in a health-promoting environment such as the waiting room.

## The building and grounds of the practice

Frequently overlooked as a health-promoting environment, the surrounding gardens, building or even practice car park present an important opportunity for communication and support. This is an environment rarely overlooked by commercial advertisers and one we should not overlook as public health practitioners. A simple noticeboard in front of the practice can be an important source of information, education and referral for the passing community. Posters can be displayed here, along with resource and referral lists, and news about useful community groups or events that promote health for people living with loss or life-threatening illness.

The grounds of the practice can also be suggested as a site for certain groups to locate themselves on special health promotion days, such as World AIDS Day, or days that promote awareness of cancer, motor neurone disease or dementia. Churches, schools and sporting clubs have used their street fronts for these purposes for years, and there is no reason (barring council regulations) that the street front of your practice could not be occasionally and gainfully employed for this purpose.

## The wider community

Probably the most difficult and time-consuming community development activity that a lone practitioner can be involved in is actually participating in community activities away from the practice. An annual school visit is possible for some but not all practitioners, especially those with a heavy case load. Few practitioners can afford to leave their practice for half a morning to record some talkback at the local radio station. Few have the confidence to write an occasional, let alone regular, article for the local newspaper. But there are other options that do allow you to engage in these activities or to promote them without leaving your office.

Some simple phone calls to the local school explaining the health promotion benefits of greater awareness around grief and loss or living with serious illness will generally be met with understanding and sympathy, if not empathy. One can suggest running a short story competition at the local school about some of these issues and volunteer to be one of a panel of judges. Poster competitions at schools also attract interest and can be promoted by the school with your help.

Although you may not have the confidence to write articles for the local newspaper, you may be able to offer a Q&A column – a question and answer service for the readers of the newspaper on matters to do with loss, care, life-threatening illness or death. Other colleagues can share the questions, and a small paragraph answer takes little time. This process can also apply to the local radio station, where pre-recorded answers can be supplied to listener questions once a week. You only have to supply a taped answer or perhaps a five-minute piece of advice or commentary.

If you are interested in and skilled at assembling web sites, then you can place useful and interesting information about a whole range of topics there and refer local agencies to this site for information, referral or advice. For local churches and temples, one can offer contact with the local bereavement or palliative care service. You can also contact the local community health service and ask what health-promoting palliative care provisions they are making for those with life-threatening illness or others living with loss. These are useful places of initial contact and dialogue, and are not necessarily time consuming.

## Final reflections

For every activity you participate in, for every interesting idea you have for health or death education, and for every environment you manipulate in the service of increasing community support for those with serious illness, loss or care issues, you need to ask yourself: 'Are these public health practices or simply diverting and novel interventions of dubious value?'. More specifically, you need to ask yourself seven important public health questions about your community practice:[2]

1. In what ways do they *prevent* social difficulties relating to death, dying, loss or care?
2. In what ways do they *harm-minimize* difficulties that we may not be able to prevent relating to death, dying, loss or care?
3. In what ways can these activities be understood as *early interventions* along the journey of death, dying, loss or care?
4. In what ways do these activities alter or *change a setting or environment* for the better in terms of our present responses to death, dying, loss or care?
5. In what ways are the proposed activities *participatory* – borne, partnered and nurtured by community members?
6. How *sustainable* will these activities or programs be without your future input?
7. How will you *evaluate* their success or usefulness so that you can justify their presence, your effort and ongoing support?

A credible public health initiative should be able to convince others and yourself that you *can* satisfactorily answer one of the first three questions. And you should be able to provide convincing responses to all questions from 4 to 7. This checklist is your personal guide to developing activities that meet all the essential health-promotion guidelines that have been and continue to be developed in all other health areas. Health-promoting palliative care is no different in its criteria for success and credibility.

The fundamental practice challenge of health promotion is to develop the often-difficult individual task of contributing to changes in the wider social environment that enhance health protection and safety. Often these contributions are not as simple as recommending a treatment or providing a piece of advice.

Health promotion is part mutual learning with the patient; part civic engagement to promote a better, more supportive interpersonal world; and part trusting yourself to be led by the patient's social, psychological or spiritual needs that take you beyond the confines of your individual practice. In these ways, health-promoting palliative care enhances the public health of those living with life-threatening illness or loss and strengthens the skills and resources of the rest of us to assist them in this complex task.

## References

1 Kellahear A. *Health Promoting Palliative Care.* Melbourne: Oxford University Press; 1999.

2 Kellehear A. *Compassionate Cities: public health and end-of-life care.* London: Routledge; 2005.

3 Baum F. *The New Public Health: an Australian perspective.* Melbourne: Oxford University Press; 1998.

4 Kellehear A. Grief and loss: past, present and future. *Med J Aust.* 2002; **177**: 176–7.

5 Kellehear A. *Dying of Cancer: the final year of life.* Chur: Harwood Academic Publishers; 1990.

6 Fawzy FI, Fawzy NW, Arndt LA, *et al.* Critical review of psychosocial interventions in cancer care. *Arch Gen Psychiatry.* 1995; **52**: 100–13.

7 Masudomi I, Isse K, Uchiyama M, *et al.* Self help groups reduce mortality risk: a 5 year follow-up study of alcoholics in the Tokyo metropolitan area. *Psychiatry Clin Neurosci.* 2004; **58**: 551–7.

8 Hildingh C, Fridlund B. A 3 year follow up of participants in peer support groups after a cardiac event. *Eur J Cardiovasc Nurs.* 2004; **3**: 315–20.

9 Campbell HS, Phaneuf MR, Deane K. Cancer peer support groups: do they work? *Patient Educ Counsel.* 2004; **55**: 3–15.

10 Barbato M. *Caring for the Dying.* Sydney: McGraw-Hill; 2002.

11 Vafiadis P. *Mutual Care in Palliative Medicine: a story of doctors and patients.* Sydney: McGraw-Hill; 2001.

12 Edgar L, Remmer J, Rosberger Z, *et al.* An oncology volunteer support organization: the benefits and fit within the health care system. *Psychooncology.* 1996; **5**: 331–41.

13 Fobair P. Cancer support groups and group therapies: Part 1: historical and theoretical background and research on effectiveness. *J Psychosoc Oncol.* 1997; **15**: 63–81.

14 Semple CJ, Sullivan K, Dunwoody L, *et al.* Psychosocial interventions for patients with head and neck cancer: past, present and future. *Cancer Nurs.* 2004; **27**: 434–41.

15 Thorman S. *A Journey Through Self-help: an evaluation of self-help in Western Australia.* Perth: Western Institute of Self Help; 1987.

# CHAPTER 9

# Summary and conclusions

*GEOFFREY MITCHELL*

We trust that this book has highlighted how the generalist skills of the family physician can be harnessed to provide truly whole-patient care in a patient's final illness. The patient-centered clinical method allows the family practitioner to engage the patient in healthcare decision-making. By being an active participant in the process, it is likely that the patient will maximize the opportunities to live their remaining life to the full.

The patient-centered clinical method has six elements:

- exploring both the disease and the illness experience
- understanding the whole person
- finding common ground
- incorporating illness and health promotion
- enhancing the patient–clinician relationship
- being realistic.

## Exploring the disease and the illness experience

In Chapter 2, Jonathon Koffman, Richard Harding and Irene Higginson provide an epidemiological basis for the importance of the book. They raise questions of equity of access, and focus on the current provision of palliative care for several marginalized groups in society. This chapter is a wake-up call to the health profession to do more to offer care to all.

In Chapter 3 David Currow and Amy Abernethy give a succinct view of the process of dying. They highlight that while life-limiting illnesses may start as one of a myriad of diseases, a 'final common pathway' is reached as multiple organs fail simultaneously. They describe what this pathway looks like, and examine what can be reversed and what cannot. They also examine the clinical picture of several common symptoms. Their chapter concludes by offering clear answers to common questions from patients about the dying process.

David and Clare Seamark explore the patient's experience of illness in Chapter 4. By contrasting real stories of the progression towards death of two patients – one with cancer and one with both cancer and chronic obstructive pulmonary disease – they place the reader alongside the patient, allowing them to understand the struggles that ensue. Jenny Hynson then describes the unique case of the dying child, offering insights into how the practitioner can help the patient along their much-shortened journey.

## Understanding the whole person

In the first part of Chapter 5, Judith Murray and Geoff Mitchell offer a framework to help understanding of the losses a patient suffers, and how the patient reacts to those losses. In the second part of the chapter Jenny Hynson again looks at the unique and tragic circumstances of the parent who must care for a dying child . Finally, the third part examines the responses of adults who care for adult relatives who are dying.

## Finding common ground

Two clinical experts, Janet Hardy and Patsy Yates, provide an overview of the treatments available for common symptoms in palliative care in Chapter 6. They emphasize that treatment involves negotiation with the person, that care of their near relatives and friends is important, and that care starts when symptom control becomes necessary – not when curative treatment fails. Importantly, they highlight that many effective treatments are not medicines, but involve education, physical and psychological therapies.

## Enhancing the patient–clinician relationship

Chapter 7 introduces Tom, a 21-year-old man dying of melanoma, and describes several aspects of his relationship with Dr Stephen Barclay. It describes the richness of the relationship experienced by Tom, his parents and Stephen. The chapter concludes with some sobering thoughts about the changing face of primary palliative care, and how these challenges might be addressed.

## Incorporating prevention and health promotion

In Chapter 8 Allan Kellehear shows how the seemingly contradictory concepts of health promotion and palliative care come together. Heath promotion is relevant in that efforts to promote well-being and prevent adverse consequences are exceedingly important in this setting. Five central tenets of health promotion are examined to show how relevant they are: prevention, harm reduction, community participation, health and death education, and social supports. He outlines how these can be enacted in a family practice setting.

Overall, the book provides an intellectual framework for the conduct of patient-centered palliative care. As such, it will be of use to those planning health services around the end of life, as well as to health administrators, teachers and practitioners. Health practitioners who are not doctors will benefit from the book, because the patient-centered clinical method is a universal template for good patient care.

# Index